Being in the Way

Being in the Way

by

Douglas Munns
VRD, BA, LDS RCS Eng

Bound Biographies

Dedication

Ron, for all his counsel, friendship
and support over so many years.

Acknowledgements

To my family and friends
and to all those listed in the appendix.

Contents

Appendices

Illustrations

Introduction

This publication is not only an outline of our family history, but also my autobiography. I have tried to relate personal experiences to some of the many developments in technology that have occurred during the lifetimes of our families, and to show how these have affected the lives of each one of us. In order to provide continuity from the past to the present it has been found necessary to include abridged versions of material from my previous publication, *Munns*, in which I attempt to outline events in my own life. Once again it has not been found possible to describe events in true chronological order, as this would have created a narrative that was far less interesting and possibly incoherent.

I often wonder whether the writer of one of the choruses that was often sung in Sunday schools, bible classes, at beach missions and elsewhere, appreciated the full implications of the words:

Yesterday, today, forever, Jesus is the same,
All may change, but Jesus never.

What changes there have been! Even those born fifty years ago cannot relate to the lack of modern facilities and the hardships experienced by their forebears. They do not understand why we cannot use much of the modern technology which they consider to be vital to modern day living.

I am grateful to the many people who made comments on my last publication and to both them and the numerous officials of libraries, family history societies and similar organisations, for their patience and for their replies to my many enquiries, and also for suggesting to me helpful prints and publications. Details of these will be found in the appendices at the end of this book.

The Munns Family

The River Thames has always played an important part in our family. Although I am not a Cockney (born within hearing of Bow Bells), I was born within the sound of the bells of *Mortlake Brewery* (which rang every morning to bring the employees to work), situated on the banks of the Thames opposite the finishing post of the annual varsity boat race (Oxford versus Cambridge). I lived in this borough until I was 14 when we moved to Hinchley Wood/Thames Ditton, once again close to the Thames.

During the summer months we often went by pleasure paddle steamer from Richmond to Hampton Court. I was at school in Richmond until I was nine, when I went to the City of London School near Blackfriars on the Victoria Embankment. Throughout the London blitz I was a part-time air raid precautions (ARP) warden in Leytonstone, very close to London Docks, and then later in life we owned a small pleasure craft moored on the Thames.

When they married in 1915, my father, Harold Munns, and my mother, Florence Mohr, made their first home close to the Thames in Surrey. I suppose this was not surprising as both their families lived near the river's banks at Erith, Kent, and many of my father's ancestors had depended on the river for their livelihood. They came from a long line of Thames Watermen and Lightermen, all of whom had served their five- to seven-year apprenticeship afloat on the Thames from as early as the age of 14, often with senior members of their family, before they received their 'Articles' from the *City of London Livery Company of Watermen*.

The earliest available record is of Thomas Munns who was articled to another by the name of Thomas Munns on 23rd September 1720. He received his freedom on 4th April 1740 which made it a very long apprenticeship. The names of many of the past members of the family appear on these records during the 19th century; my great grandfather had five sons, all of whom served their apprenticeship on Thames barges, although not all continued in this trade.

In the 19th century Erith became a very important town on the southern bank of the Thames because upstream the river became very shallow between there and Woolwich. As a result, many ships either off-loaded all their cargo at Erith, or at least reduced it, so that they could proceed further upstream. This brought considerable prosperity to the town, as well as keeping it in touch with many of the events in the mainstream of national and international history. It was even proposed that a ship canal should be built between Woolwich and Erith to make it easier for shipping to sail up to central London, but this plan was eventually abandoned because of the cost involved.

Following the opening of the railway from London Bridge to Erith in 1849, several manufacturing firms moved to the area. Amongst these were *Fraser and Chalmers* where my father was employed as an office boy when he left school at the age of 13. He continued his education at night school which enabled him eventually to join the firm of *Watts Fincham & Company*, engineering buyers, in the City of London. *Callender Cables & Conductors* opened a factory in 1896 and my Auntie Cissie joined this firm as a draughtswoman after she left school. *Vicker, Sons & Maxim*, ordnance manufacturers of Sheffield, opened a branch in Erith at about the same time, and my mother's father joined this firm when the family moved from Birmingham to Northumberland Heath; family records suggest that he was actively involved in the development of the machine-gun.

Before the railways were built, the Thames was the main thoroughfare for transporting goods in and out of London, including those commodities that were arriving by ship from all parts of the world. Barges, sailing and man-propelled, were built to cope with this trade. My grandfather was articled to his father and enjoyed a very successful career on the river, eventually owning his own sailing barge. This was even before the age of steam when ships from all over the world docked in London, some of their cargo being off-loaded onto these sailing barges for onward transportation to their final destination. This could be to one of

18

the London Thames-side warehouses, to the River Medway, across the English Channel to near continental ports, or along the Grand Union canal.

Many of these sailing barges were built in one of the numerous shipbuilding yards on the River Medway and my grandfather's ship, *Nina*, was no exception. She was built in the yard of *Gill & Sons* of Strood in 1884 and was known as a 'stumpy sailing barge', being of shallow draught so that she could enter the Regent's Canal and other similar shallow canals (compared with the Thames). She was registered until 31st March 1923, but we have been unable to find her history after that date. Details of her registration and her specifications can be seen in the Appendix.

My grandfather and his family lived in various properties in Erith. In 1881 they were living in Crayford Road, and then in 1897, in Maxinfield Road. In the early 1900s they had built, with the help of his wife's family who were builders in Bexleyheath, two semi-detached houses in Bexley Road, Northumberland Heath, where they lived in No74. One of his sons inherited this property after his parents died and was still living in it at the outbreak of World War II.

I never really knew much about my grandfather's life as I was only twelve when he died of myocardial degeneration in 1932. We visited his home two or three times a year for a cup of tea when we were staying with my other grandmother who lived nearby. The house had a rather dark front parlour where his wife used to sit in a rocking chair wrapped in a shawl. There was also a large pedal organ in the room. At the rear of the house there was a long garden with an orchard at the far end, a wooden shed/greenhouse and a swing. I can well remember when my grandfather built me a wooden model sailing yacht for my eighth or ninth birthday and we sailed this on Penn Ponds in Richmond Park.

Shortly after his 80th birthday (it must have been around 1920) my grandfather, who had started work on the water at the age of five, retired and was interviewed by a reporter from the local weekly newspaper. After saying that my grandfather was a healthy and vigorous man the report continues:

> He loves the water so much that he goes out in his
> rowing boat every day. To use his own words, he

"knows every inlet of the old river from Sheerness to Shepperton" and is to be seen nearly every day down by the waterside. He spoke of the lost loveliness of the river bank at Erith. "They were the days," said the veteran reflectively, "when 60 or 70 yachts lay off Erith, and later the foreign, as well as the English paddle boat, could be seen any day from the shore. There weren't any screw steamers then. I began work as a cabin boy at five on my father's boat and I began to earn money at the age of nine, five shillings a week."

Mr Munns belongs to Erith's oldest water-going family. His father and his grandfather were watermen and he believes his great grandfather was in the same line of business. Early rising and plenty of fresh air is Mr Munns' old-age recipe, and it looks as though Erith is going to have a centenarian waterman one of these days. "I remember when the diamond boats, such as *Sea Swallow* and the like, ran between London and Gravesend and called at Erith," he reminisced. "In the summer they went to Sheerness. In those days there was no coal wharf at *Cory's* but there used to be a line along which horses drew trucks - that was where the *Co-operative Stores* stand now. The *Pier Hotel* stood where *Cory's* offices are now and lower down were the yachts owned by many titled people. At the Round House, Anchor Bay, lived the captain of the old *Eagle*. I was born at the back of where the *Cross Keys* now is. There used to be a right of way through there leading to what was called Martin's shore, a nice place. I recall a huge French yacht being built at Erith; it stretched right across the beautiful Erith gardens, a popular place with many visitors in the district. Boats which afterwards went to Khartoum were also made at Erith.

"In course of time I became my father's mate and went on the barge *Arthur*. I remember when the *Royal London Yacht Club* held their meeting at the *Crown Hotel*. I used to love sailing, as I do now, and I have had numerous adventures. Once a huge anchor fell from a steamship and sunk my barge; I was thrown into the water but escaped. Another time I was swept into the water at night by a whirling rope. For 39 years I owned my own barge and slept on the water pretty often. I still go out regularly now and I often think of the old days on the river at Erith. In these days of six- and seven-thousand-ton vessels at Erith it is strange to recall the tiny ones that once anchored there. Last winter a 10,000-tonner was off Erith!"

He also witnessed one of the greatest tragedies on the Thames involving a pleasure steamer. In early September 1878 the *Princess Alice*, a twin-paddle pleasure steamer, was returning from a daytrip from London to Rosherville Gardens near Gravesend when, near North Woolwich Pier, a much larger vessel, the steam collier *Bywell Castle*, hit her amidships splitting the vessel into two halves. She sank within minutes and many hundreds of lives were lost. As a result of this accident, navigation regulations on the Thames and other inland waterways were introduced.

* * * * *

My grandparents had six children, three boys and three girls, my father being the youngest. One of the girls, Ethel, died in 1893 from tuberculosis at the age of 16 and one of the sons died in 1920 from tetanus contracted as the result of a motorcycle accident. Alice, a schoolteacher, married Horace Herbert Gill in 1905. Edie, also a schoolteacher, married John Charles Martin in 1907. Herbert, a fitter, married Bessie Maker in 1917 and Harold, my father, an engineer's buyer, married Florence Mohr in 1915.

Many of the Munns' families were members of the Erith Avenue Road Congregational Church and a retired minister of that church, the Rev Moses Williams, with whom my grandfather formed a close friendship, conducted his funeral service at the Erith cemetery on Saturday 27th February 1932. One of my grandfather's brothers, George, and one of my grandmother's relatives, Mr W.R.C. Smith, were deacons. Alice, my grandfather's daughter, was actively engaged with the Avenue Sunday School Band of Hope and from their minutes it would appear that one of her responsibilities was the children's choir.

My father was born at Erith, Kent on the 18th April 1887. He attended the local Board School and in the 1901 census, when he was 13, his profession is recorded as office boy! At that time the family were living next door to Erith vicarage where George Adams, the vicar of my mother's church, lived. Assuming that my father was a member of the Band of Hope in his church, and we know that my mother belonged to this organisation in her church, perhaps this is how they first met. In 1911 he was employed in the shipping department of *Fraser & Chalmers Ltd*, a major employer in the district. They also had offices in the City of London at London Wall near to where my father was to work for the next thirty years. His final reference from *Frasers* stated that he was a 'painstaking and industrious clerk'.

I have already mentioned that after leaving school my father attended night classes and he gained, amongst others, certificates in shorthand and book-keeping. After leaving *Frasers* he joined *Watts, Fincham & Company*, a firm of engineer buyers, in Billiter Street in the City of London, and was employed there until he was made redundant during the depression in the early 1930s. Their offices on the second floor were very dark and dingy and there was an ancient self-operated lift without post-World War II safety devices.

In 1908 a new unit of the 4th Home Counties (Howitzer) Brigade, Royal Field Artillery (Territorial Force) was formed in Erith at Trevethan, Bexley Road. My father and his friends joined this unit, a mounted unit with the field guns that are still used at ceremonial occasions. He was presumably in a reserved occupation when war was declared in 1914 as he did not go to France with this unit. In September 1916, however, he joined the Royal Naval Air Service in the Writer/Stores branch and was stationed at Crystal Palace and Wandsworth, also serving in France at Luxeuil Air Station. Before being discharged on the cessation of hostilities, he had passed the Petty Officer promotion examination.

Our family moved from the flat in Cromwell Place, Mortlake Green, where I was born, to another rented property, a semi-detached house in Palewell Park, East Sheen. This was in 1920/21 and several years later my father purchased a newly built house at 64 Richmond Park Road, a road leading up from the main Upper Richmond Road to Sheen Gate, Richmond Park. He had to obtain a mortgage to enable him to do this but, as was always his intention, redeemed it at an early date, fortunately before he was made redundant. The spare ground at the rear of this property was developed as the Sheen House Hard Court Tennis Club, of which my father became a director and honorary secretary.

Following his redundancy, he looked for a cheaper property which resulted in our moving to a detached house in Hinchley Wood (*Luxeuil*, 108 Manor Road North), property being much cheaper in this developing part of Surrey at the end of the newly constructed Kingston-By-Pass. We lived here until, due to dwindling capital, he was forced to sell it in the summer of 1939, a few weeks before war was declared. Uncle Horace kindly offered us a first floor flat in one of his properties in Leytonstone, East London, a few miles from the London docks. This was a very basic, two bedroom property with no proper bathroom and poor kitchen facilities, but with no money in the bank we were lucky to have a roof over our heads - 'beggars cannot be choosers'. We managed living in this property until an unexploded bomb landed outside during the London blitz, by which time my father was up in Kirkby, Lancashire, and soon my mother joined him there. I went to live with John Ruff and his mother in Carshalton, Surrey, remaining there until I joined the Royal Navy in 1942.

Following the devastating blow of redundancy, my father tried, with the help of funds from his brother-in-law, my Uncle Horace, to set-up his own business, *Munns Gill and Company*, as middle-men in the engineering trade. The business failed as so many of his old colleagues were also badly affected by the depression and could not offer him business. However, war clouds were on the horizon and the government had issued instructions that firms were to build air raid shelters for their employees. My father was appointed the south London representative of one of the firms supplying such industrial shelters.

When war was declared in 1939, a Ministry of Supply (MoS) was established and my father was successful in being appointed as Chief Stores Manager, a responsible job entailing close cooperation with the managers of other departments at a newly built Royal Ordinance factory at Kirkby about eight miles to the north-east of Liverpool. Although he was not given one of the newly built manager's houses in the office complex, he was given a much better requisitioned farmhouse just outside the northern boundary of the site within about a ten-minute cycle ride of the main factory entrance. When the factory was closed down at the end of the war he moved to one of the London MoS offices near St Paul's Cathedral, where he was responsible for organising the disposal of all types of war materials no longer required by the government. My mother continued to live in the old farmhouse at Kirby whilst my father stayed with relations in London.

* * * * *

When I arrived in the UK for demob on a troopship from Singapore where our hospital ship *HMHS Gemsalemme* was then stationed, my father was on the dockside at Southampton to greet me and, after staying in Kirby for a few weeks with my mother, I took up an appointment in Norman Gray's dental practice in Eastbourne. There was hardly any property available anywhere in the UK, but eventually I found a flat in this town and my mother was able to leave Kirkby and we were together as a family again (even though my father had to travel to London each day). When I left Eastbourne for a practice in the City of London, we continued living in this flat with both myself and my father travelling to London each day. Then one evening I received a telephone call from my friend and fellow dental surgeon, Raymond Bird, with the news that a flat had become vacant in the block of flats where he lived, but the landlord needed to know immediately if we would like it. Thus we moved to Cockfosters.

My father could not afford to buy a house but as soon as I was earning a reasonable salary, and with the help of a mortgage, I was able to purchase a semi-detached family home in the same district. He was retired in 1952 at the age of 65 but unfortunately his short wartime employment with the MoS did not entitle him to a government pension. He was fortunate in finding part-time employment where he was responsible for organising the wages of a small firm in Waltham Abbey, but lack of finances continued to be a problem.

When we were living in Malvern in the 1960s I managed to find my mother and father a flat in the town and so, with some support from the Freemasons, they moved and we sold the house in Cockfosters. My father had been a mason for most of his adult life and must have been initiated before the outbreak of World War I (I suspect shortly after he joined *Watts, Fincham & Co*) as he received the Masonic medal, given to all those masons who served in HM Forces during The Great War. He held various offices in The Lodge of St James, including officiating at instruction classes on Monday evenings during the winter months in the 20s and 30s. He was installed as Worshipful Master in 1939.

My father died suddenly in Malvern in 1979 at the age of 92. His funeral took place at Worcester crematorium and was attended by family and friends.

The Mohr Family

My maternal great grandfather, Carl Gustav Mohr, was born in Coblenz, Prussia, in 1833 and emigrated to the UK in 1854. Why he came to England we do not know, but it has been suggested that it was to avoid conscription into the Prussian army. My mother had a medal, the Prussian 'Kriegsdenkmonze' (war memorial medal) dated 1813/1814, which she said was earned by his father. (*See Appendix*)

In 1868, my great grandfather was granted British citizenship. He was at this time living in Stratford Street, Camp Hill, Birmingham and was in partnership with George Edward Servis, a wire maker and birdcage manufacturer, their works being in Bolton Road, Small Heath, Birmingham. Over the course of his life, my great grandfather registered many inventions with the patent office. The one which was probably most appreciated was a gear case for ladies bicycles, designed to ensure that the ladies long skirts and dresses were not soiled from an oily chain. A list of his patents, and details of this particular patent, can be found in the appendices.

On 22nd December 1860 he married Clara Chatwin Duddell in Birmingham. They had eleven children amongst whom were Gustav, who emigrated to the USA; Louis Ernest my grandfather; Clara Chatwin (Auntie Clara) and Florence Minnie whom I knew as Auntie Florrie. My great grandfather lived with Auntie Florrie at 27 Wilton Road, Sparkhill, Birmingham, for many years after his wife died.

My great grandfather was well over 90 when he visited us in East Sheen, yet he walked from there to Richmond each day. It was in Richmond, at an antique shop, that he bought a Jacobean hall bench (called a settle) for my mother, thinking it would go nicely in our hall and complement the old family oak coffer - it did, but left little room in the small hallway! After he returned to Birmingham he sent me the first station for my model railway. My mother and I often visited Auntie Florrie after his death and I well remember that the midday meal was never served before 4.00 pm, often later. Whilst there, we used to visit other family relations.

Shortly before my mother's 100th birthday, she wrote the following based on her own memories and those of previous generations of her family:

> In the year 1882 Sarah Ann Dale, a young girl of 18 years, left her home in Tarring, near Worthing, Sussex, for the start of her journey to Australia, the journey in those days of sailing ships taking some eight months. Her brothers had preceded her in order to build a house for their parents. The first house was burnt down before it was completed. Their mother did not arrive at this new home as she was taken from the ship in Sydney to hospital where she died. Sometime after that her grandfather joined them and would have returned to England with my mother's family but he was then turned 80 and almost blind.
>
> In about 1883, a young man, Louis Ernest Mohr, left his home in Birmingham to settle in Australia. He eventually met Sarah and they married. They were my parents.
>
> I do not know much about my mother's family, except that they were a very old English family and her father ran a business making riding boots for the gentry of that period. He must have retired early to enable him to join his family in Australia. Grandfather Dale was Chief Superintendent of the Thames Police and retired to Torquay, leaving for Australia after his wife died. One of my mother's brothers was a bandmaster in Sydney. Because of some disagreement, their youngest brother walked out of the house when he was 15 and was never seen again.
>
> My father was born in Birmingham in 1863, the second of a family of eleven children - eight sons and three daughters. He was 21 when he emigrated to

28

Australia and, after his marriage at Pitt Street Congregational Church, Sydney, moved to Camden, a township on the edge of the bush and on the banks of the River Murray about 40 miles from Sydney. One of my sisters and myself were born there, the family eventually returning to England when I was three or four years old.

My father's family, on the male side, were associated with the Duke of Argyll (Campbell clan). The Scottish clans were always fighting and used to go over to the continent to fight the French and Germans. Evidently some of my father's forebears married German women and settled there. One ancestor of the Mohr family was an interpreter to Frederick the Great. He was married to Baroness Lowensteen who was a Baroness in her own right.

Another ancestor, Joseph Mohr, wrote the words of the carol *Silent Night, Holy Night*. He had been ordained by the Bishop of Saltzburg on August 21st 1815. When he later went to the church of St Nicholas, Oberndorf to prepare for a Christmas Mass, he found that the organ would not work - it seems that mice had gnawed holes in the bellows! The organist was a schoolmaster called Gruber who also played the guitar. Concerned that Christmas Mass must not be dull, he composed music to suit Joseph's words and, with this guitar accompaniment, they both sang the new carol.

Joseph Mohr died on 4th November 1848. In 1899, St Nicholas Church was unfortunately destroyed by floods, but a memorial chapel was built on the same site in which there is a bronze relief to the memory of both Gruber and Mohr. The local mayor, priest, and villagers place flowers on it each anniversary to commemorate those who gave such a lovely carol to the world. This information was passed on to me by my uncle through my grandfather. The first English version of this carol was made by Miss Emily S Elliott in 1858, for the choir of St Mark's Church, Brighton. The old organ is now in a museum in Salzburg.

Both my parents were well read and a great help to us children. My father was very strict, but we enjoyed a lot of fun with him. He and his elder brother went to King Edward Grammar School, Birmingham, and they finished their education in Koblenz, Germany.

My father invented the technique for shooting down the zeppelins in World War I, but he never received recognition for this by the firm with whom he worked. One of his brothers, Uncle Max, sang in the choir at Manchester Cathedral. Another brother, Uncle Oliver, was a Shakespearian actor (professional name Richard Harries). Uncle Stanley was a stained glass window artist and designed a window for Belfast Cathedral. We saw this window when it was displayed at the Wembley Exhibition.

Auntie Clara was a professional singer. At first she worked for her father in his office for the magnificent sum of 6d per week, and with this she was able to take singing lessons. She eventually joined the Birmingham Repertoire. One of my sisters, Cissie, was an artist, and another, Ethel, wrote a lot of poetry, even sending some poems to King George VI. (*See Appendix*) Uncle Fred was also an artist and designed china for a Staffordshire firm (*Daltons*, I think). As a family we were also very musical but never gained fame!

* * * * *

One always hopes that oral tradition will be supported by historical fact, but unfortunately this is not always the case. Although two of my grandmother's brothers were educated at King Edward's School, Birmingham, we know that my mother's father was educated at Sparkbrook Middle Class School, Stratford Road, Birmingham (headmaster E J Reynolds, G.C.M.), and on the 23rd December 1869, was awarded a prize for drawing. I am grateful to researchers at the Theatre Museum in London, the university libraries in both Birmingham and Bristol, and the Birmingham

Conservatoire Information Services Library, for researching other family members with alleged acting and singing talents, although without results. One problem, of course, is that we do not know whether they performed under stage names, but it seems they were probably amateurs rather than professionals.

The narrative of *Silent Night* would seem to be true and there is a museum in Salzburg devoted to the history of this well-known carol, although there is no evidence that Josef Mohr was a direct relative of my mother's family. As he was a catholic priest, he would have been celibate and therefore having no family and, according to the curator of the Kelten Museum, Hallem, no illegitimate children are known. It is, of course, always possible that mother's great grandfather was a brother. Details of Joseph Mohr's various appointments as a priest are to be found in the Konsistotial Archiv of the Archivdiocese in Salzburg.

* * * * *

It has proved impossible to trace any connection with a Scottish clan, although families in the 16th and 17th centuries moved freely between the UK and the continent. In state papers written in 1693 during the reign of William and Mary, it is recorded that a pass was issued to 'Peter Mohr to go to Harwich and Holland'. Other papers, dated 1695, give permission for 'Lieutenant William Mohr and one servant to go to Harwich or Gravesend for Holland'. In the 1800s, *The Times* reports on musical concerts being given in Hanover Square Rooms by musicians from Germany, with a Mr Mohr playing the flute.

My mother's father did arrive in Australia in 1883. 'It is almost beyond comprehension to realise the dangers and trauma these pioneer settlers had to overcome', writes the author of an article in the 1890 edition of the King Edward's school chronicle. He describes the horrific experiences of one of the old boys on a sailing ship bound for Australia towards the end of the 19th century, a voyage taking many months. They only sighted land once on the whole voyage, and then it was off the coast of Brazil. How the vessel got there is, the author writes, 'an unfathomable mystery… the weather they experienced was eccentric in the extreme - at one time the saloon was swamped and they were nearly washed out of their berths, but at another, owing to calms and contrary winds, they advanced at the alarming rapidity of two miles a day!'

With such travelling conditions, it seems highly probable that my grandmother's mother either sustained some injury or developed an illness that resulted in her death in hospital shortly after arriving in Australia. The writer concludes, however, that, 'there is a future for those going to Australia, a country of nearly a million square miles inhabited by about 40,000 white people - a country one quarter the area of the whole of Europe with a population no larger than that of Edgbaston'.

Shortly after my mother's father arrived in Sydney, he set up business as a marble mason at 19 Selwyn Street, Moore Park, (*see Appendix*) specialising as a chimney piece and marble fender maker, and a shop fitter. He also repaired and polished all kinds of marble work. On 25th September 1886, he married Sarah Ann Dale at Pitt Street Congregational Church, Sydney. Shortly after that they moved to Camden where he opened an ironmongers shop and also undertook various projects in people's homes. My mother was born on 3rd July 1889 and her sister, Alice (Cissie), about one year later. Her mother had had a baby before either of them was born but she died when only a few months old.

My mother and her sister, together with their mother and father, returned to the UK in 1891 on the *Orient Line* steamship *RMS Prizaba*, arriving in London on Christmas Eve, a much more pleasant journey than when their father was outward bound on a sailing vessel. They settled in the Sparkhill area of Birmingham where her other three sisters, Agnes, Ethel and Stella, and brother Arthur, were born (there was another brother, Louis Ernest, but he died when only 11 weeks old). My mother attended the Oakley Road Infants School, Formans Lane, Birmingham, and received a prize for good attendance whilst there.

When her father was successful in gaining an appointment at *Vicars Engineering Works*, Erith, Kent, the family moved to Northumberland Heath, firstly to a house in Hengist Road and then to Horsa Road. This was a small semi-detached house at the end of a terrace with a parlour at the front, a kitchen/scullery at the rear downstairs and two double and one single bedroom upstairs. There was an outside toilet but no bathroom, just a copper for boiling water and a tin bath in the scullery. It was not until the 1920s that the upper rear bedroom was altered to accommodate a small bathroom and toilet at the rear, although one still had to walk through the single room to get to this bathroom.

My mother then attended Brook Street School before moving on to Picardy Girl's School. After leaving school she became a companion to an elderly lady living nearby and attended evening classes, gaining Pitman certificates in shorthand and typing.

When my mother's sister Cissie left school, she obtained a job as a draughtswoman at *Callendar Cables*, Erith. She had a very interesting career with this firm, not only in her own department, but also preparing illustrated addresses for retiring personnel and for other special occasions. She was eventually promoted to the firm's head office in London in the early '30s and was then able to purchase a small bungalow in Bexleyheath (11 Francis Avenue, Kent) for herself and her mother. She also attended various evening classes in drawing, painting, and woodwork.

Agnes became a nanny and spent many years on a sheep ranch some 500 miles north of Sydney, New South Wales, owned by the Bernard-Stewart's, a Scottish family. She brought several of their children into the world. When they had returned to the UK, she attended many of their family functions, including weddings of her previous charges, and later she was asked to help with their families. During the intervening years, she served as nanny to a family in Kenya.

Ethel had a chequered childhood and spent many years in and out of hospitals, firstly in the Birmingham Children's Hospital and then King's College Hospital, London, after the family moved to Kent. She had some infection of one of her legs (TB?) and wore a calliper for many years. This illness interfered with her schooling, but she also became a nanny, serving with many families, and she was a life-long member of the Girl's Friendly Society.

Stella joined the Women's Auxiliary Community Service towards the end of World War I, then sailed for India in 1920 to take up the post of secretary to the principal of Bishop Cotton School, a

Church Missionary Society (CMS) school, in Simla. In 1925 she married Angus Keith Cargill, an engineer with the Indian civil service. They had two children, Ruth and Heather. Unfortunately, Angus died suddenly and, because he worked for the Indian civil service rather than the British civil service, Stella did not receive a widow's pension. She returned to this country but the financial situation led to difficult times bringing up her two children.

Arthur was employed by a local firm in Erith and did much for the local boy scouts, becoming a district commissioner. He married Marion Dixon on 13th September 1930.

My mother attended the Sunday school at St Paul's Church, Northumberland Heath and we still have her 1908 Scripture Union card. She was confirmed by the Bishop of Rochester on 11th May 1907 and I can well remember her attending early Sunday morning communion service at Mortlake Parish Church when I was a young boy. In those days, services at Easter and at other festivals were often so crowded that she chose to attend the early service commencing at 7.00 am, although there were later similar services.

My mother was a very active member of the parish of Mortlake with East Sheen, as was the Duchess of York when she was living at White Lodge, Richmond Park, and both helped at the summer fêtes in the vicarage garden and at the Christmas fairs. The latter were held on the first floor of the Wigan Institute, North Worple Way, built in 1866 by Frederick Wigan for the people of Mortlake. She was also one of the many parishioners present on the 24th October 1928 when the Duchess of York laid the foundation stone of the new All Saints Church at the top of East Sheen Avenue. Great detail was given to the designing of this church, not only keeping it within church architectural traditions, but also to ensure the smooth running of services, particularly Holy Communion services. Another occasion at which she was present was the 50th anniversary service of this church, attended by the Queen Mother.

A life-long member of the Mother's Union (MU), my mother served on various committees and when she was living in Cockfosters, North London, in the '50s, was on the diocesan panel of speakers. She was also a great supporter of home and overseas missions, being treasurer of a working party in East Sheen in the '20s and helping with missionary exhibitions whilst there and when living in Cockfosters. She was a member of the choir at Christ Church, Cockfosters, as well as that of the Townswomen's Guild, and a member of a mandolin band in her early married life. She was also very interested in pokerwork, the craft of burning designs on wood with a heated platinum point. She was always very active in the community, with bridge and tennis being her main interests, but her family always came first, even if this meant disappointing others at times. She always took me to Sunday school, this having priority over all other engagements.

* * * * *

When war was imminent in the late '30s, both my mother and I trained as air raid wardens, the training lectures and films being partly based on the lessons learnt from air raids during the Spanish civil war. We then helped with training and organising air raid precaution examinations at the council offices in Esher, Surrey (where we were then living), and with the distribution of gasmasks in the area. Just before the outbreak of war, we had to vacate our house in Hinchley Wood, Esher, and move to a small flat in East London that left much to be desired. My mother became a full-time Warden on Post 21 in the Borough of Leyton, a very humiliating job in a very confined place - one woman amongst men who smoked heavily. Her job included responsibility for a large communal air raid shelter on Wanstead Flats. She remained in charge throughout the Battle of Britain air raids. During this period of her life she suffered much mental and spiritual anguish, added to by the fact that her husband was away from home, having been appointed as Stores Manager at ROF Kirkby, a munitions establishment near Liverpool. She eventually moved up to Kirkby herself and remained there for the duration of the war. She soon made friends there with nearby farmer's wives, with members of the MU at the local church and, through their social club, wives of my father's colleagues at the factory. She also joined their badminton club.

Because of the extensive area taken over by the government, many roads had been closed or diverted, with the result that one had to travel three to four miles to reach the village of Kirkby with its church, station, and other amenities. Mother used the rather poor train service to travel to Liverpool for her weekly duties at the Royal Naval War Library and to visit an old East Sheen family whose office had been evacuated to Wigan. Eventually the tramway from the centre of Liverpool was extended to the factory gates. They usually attended the morning service at Knowsley Church on Lord Derby's estate, because it was a shorter journey. My mother and father also made friends with the manager, and his wife, of the firm in St Helens that manufactured the specially formulated composition, not unlike that used for dental impressions, with which bombs were packed. They visitied each other's houses when petrol rations permitted.

* * * * *

Despite all the rationing restrictions and shortage of housing, life gradually returned to normal after VJ day and as soon as I was earning a regular salary I was able to rent a flat for our family, firstly in Eastbourne and then in London. Eventually I was able, with the help of a mortgage, to purchase a small semi-detached house in Cockfosters, North London. After my marriage to Beryl in 1955 we also had a second mortgage on our own house. Eventually, with a growing family, we found the strain of two mortgages too great and so, reluctantly, we found it necessary to sell the house in Cockfosters where my mother and father were still living. However, this was not before we had secured a retirement flat for them in Hill House, Malvern, Worcestershire, the town in which we were then living. They were able to pay the rent for this with help from the Freemasons and with government grants. Unfortunately a few years after they moved there my mother was knocked down by a car and fractured her hip. She never really regained full mobility.

When my father died in 1979, we were living in Godalming, Surrey, and we made preliminary enquiries for my mother regarding vacancies in Masonic establishments. Her GP, however, who visited her regularly, considered that my mother could continue to live on her own in her flat. We accepted his decision on the understanding that he would advise us when he considered she required more sheltered accommodation.

My father had been a Freemason for most of his life, so when it eventually became necessary for my mother to leave her flat, she was able to move into one of their care homes: Lord Harris Court, Sindlesham, near Reading. Here she had a large en-suite room until the last years of her life when she needed to move to their sickbay. She was then over 100 years old. The staff were very kind and understanding but, as with any establishment of this kind, the residents had various grumbles which we heard all about on our weekly visits! The chaplains were also kind and helpful but the sad thing was that the Mothers Union, and similar organisations that she had supported all her life, rarely contacted her. My father's Masonic Lodge, the Lodge of St James, always sent her a gift at Christmas.

My mother had been an avid letter writer all her life and kept up correspondence with all her friends. Their replies were always appreciated but this correspondence dwindled as everyone got older. One of the many addresses in my mother's diary was that of her cousin, Monica, who was the Prioress of the Carmelite Monastery in Wolverhampton.

Sadly the art of letter writing seems to be lost and the world is the poorer for it. In this age of electronics and computers your old friends do not seem to want to know you if you cannot exchange e-mails with them.

My mother died aged 104. Several of her relations and friends attended her funeral, conducted by a former chaplain of Lord Harris Court, at the Wokingham crematorium. Many sent gifts in her memory and these were donated to the Missions to Seamen (as it was then known). She had supported the mission from the time of my service in the Royal Navy and had been a voluntary worker in Liverpool for the naval library that provided the much needed books for those on many lonely voyages. We received many letters following her death of which this, from the chaplain who led her funeral service, is typical - 'What a wonderful Christian example she has left for all who shared her love and fellowship. My wife joins me in thankfulness for the many words of love she shared with her. Our loss is heaven's gain'.

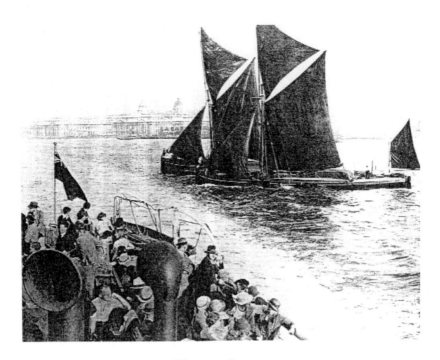

Thames Barges

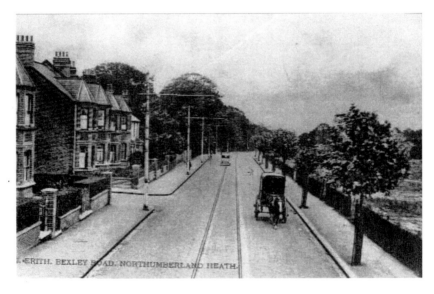

Bexley Road, Erith

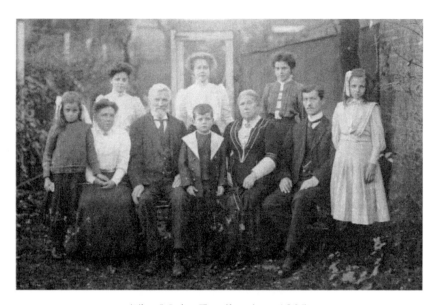

The Mohr Family, circa 1905
Back row: Agnes, Cissie, my mother
Front row: Stella, Grannie, Great-Grandpa, Arthur, Great-Grandma, Grandpa, Ethel

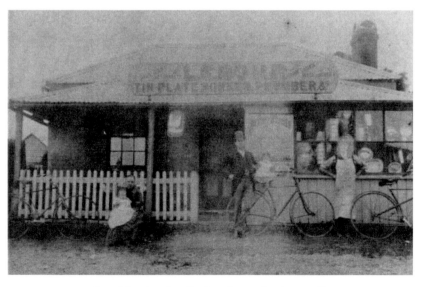

Outside the family business in Australia
Mother seated on the bicycle with her father beside her
Mother's sister Cissie on their mother's lap

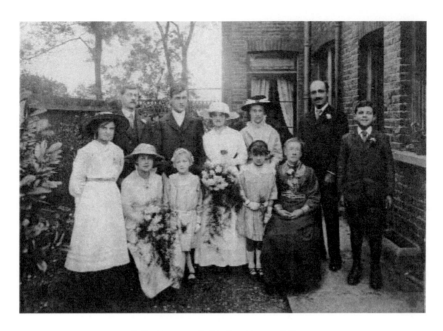

Mother and Father's wedding

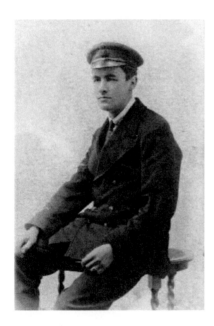

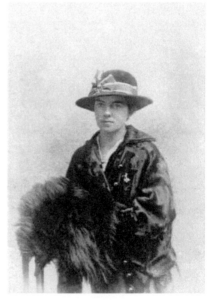

Father in his naval uniform
c1916

Mother

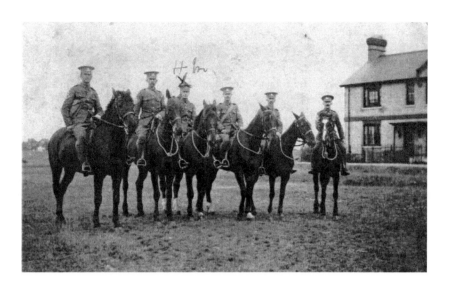

Father in the Royal Horse Artillery c1912

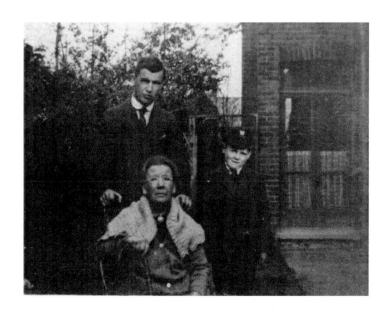

With father and Granny Munns

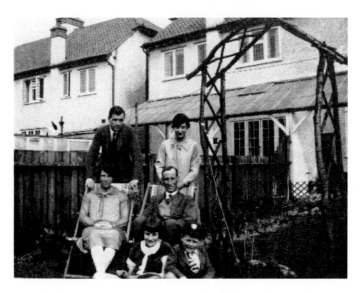

Back garden of 64 Richmond Park Road, East Sheen, 1925
Standing: My father and Cousin Kathleen
Seated: Auntie Edie and Uncle Charlie
Front: Cousin Joan and myself

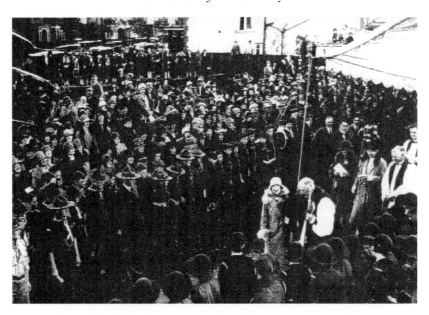

The Duchess of York laying the foundation stone
of All Saints Church, East Sheen

Early Years

I was born on 14th August 1919 at 6 Cromwell Place (Cromwell House), Mortlake, Surrey. I understand that my Aunt Agnes was present at my birth, but I have no recollection of this! I imagine that I was the first baby to be born in these flats since the end of World War I and as such, was befriended by many of the occupants.

In No3, an upper flat at the end of the terrace, lived the Misses Ada, Clara and Helen Tyrrell. Although elderly and suffering from severe arthritis, they made very fine lace. They gave several articles to my mother, including table clothes and tray clothes. I wonder whether, in their younger days, they were connected with the lace industry of the area. I best remember them because every year at Christmas, and on my birthday, they gave me a half-crown (2s.6d). Their niece was the author Mabel L. Tyrrell who is perhaps best known for her book The Secrets of Nicholas Culpepper. Nicholas Culpepper was a famous herbalist, and the book is beautifully illustrated with various herbs. She also wrote many books for children and I was sent copies of several of them - *Camilla the Cat*, *The Adventures of a Monkey* and *The Bottle of Sweets* - which I have kept to this day.

In the basement flat below ours lived Mrs Morgan and her son Cyril. He was one of my godfathers and I knew him as Uncle Cyril. My other godparents were Auntie Agnes and Uncle Thompson (whom I think was a Royal Naval Air Service [RNAS] wartime colleague of my father).

Mr and Mrs Lock (stage name Vernon) lived at number five. My memory of them is that they used to run a summer concert party at Seaford, Sussex. For two years my mother and I stayed there for a few days with Mr Lock's grandmother. We attended the show and my mother helped in the box office.

Mortlake is a place of great antiquity. To persons of my generation I suppose it is best known for its association with the annual inter-varsity boat race, but the presence of stone-age implements in the River Thames at this location suggest the existence of a prehistoric settlement. Before the Norman Conquest in the 11th century, Earl Harold owned lands and a fishery on the riverside, whilst the manor of Mortlake was occupied by the Archbishop of Canterbury. The first recorded place of worship in the village of Mortlake was a chapel erected in 1348, under licence from Edward III, and Adomar, the priest of Wimbledon, was enjoined to appoint a curate-in-charge. The chapel stood near the manor house, on the site of the present brewery, and served the spiritual needs of the villagers for nearly two hundred years.

The manor belonged to the archbishopric of Canterbury until 1536 when Archbishop Cranmer transferred it to King Henry VIII in exchange for other lands. He, in turn, arranged for a church to be built on the present site in 1543. Since then, many additions have been made to this building, including the extension of the north aisle and the reconstruction of a chancel, nave, and south aisle. The only surviving relic from the ancient chapel of Mortlake is the 15th century font, in which I was baptised on 5th October 1919 by the Rev H.W. Benson. We still have my SPCK baptismal card - 'Be thou faithful unto death and I will give thee a crown of life'.

In about 1921 we moved to 2 Palwell Park, East Sheen. This was part of a development of the fifty acre Palwell estate of farm and meadowland. It had been sold in 1896 and the development was complete by the outbreak of the First World War. Along the Upper Richmond Road there were shops with flats above, and in East Sheen Avenue, Gilpin Avenue, Park Avenue, and Palwell Park, houses. Our house was a semi-detached Victorian property, lit by gas, just around the corner from Upper Richmond Road, along which ran a frequent service of buses - 33, 37, & 73. Number 33 plied between Richmond and Waterloo Station and number 73 between Richmond and Stoke Newington. Both services were routed via Hammersmith, Kensington and Hyde Park Corner, the former also via Piccadilly and Strand and the latter via Marble Arch and Oxford Street. At weekends during the summer months some services were extended to Hampton Court, the 33 via Bushey Park and the 73 via Kingston. Number 37 plied between Twickenham (via Richmond) and Peckham (via Putney). In 1921 these were all of open top double deck stock, but it was not long before the upper deck was covered over but the external staircase remained uncovered. It was not until the end of the decade that new stock with internal staircases was introduced.

As well as these red *General Omnibus Company* buses, there were a number of 'pirate' buses, as my friend and I called them. They were run by private companies and tended to speed past the red buses, which made them very popular with us boys! They had various liveries - brown, chocolate, green, etc. Fares were 2d to Richmond, 4d to Kensington and 7d to Oxford Circus, Piccadilly and Hampton Court, with half fares for children over three.

My memories of living in Palwell Park are rather vague. I know we had two deliveries of milk each day; the early morning delivery being in a heavy metal can with a hinged lid. I dropped one of these on my big toe and the nail went black and peeled off.

Soon after we moved to East Sheen, Mick, a mixed breed wire haired terrier, joined the family. He had been a gift to Auntie Stella from her boyfriend Kenyon and she asked us to look after him when she sailed to India. He lived until the early 1930s.

Whilst living in Palwell Park, my paternal grandfather gave me a sailing boat named *Douglas*, which he had constructed himself. I was very disappointed with it because it had brown sails not white ones like those in the toyshops. The reason for the brown sails, I now know, was that many of the sailing barges on the Thames, including his own, had brown sails. I used to sail it on the ponds in Richmond Park, a wonderful place where I was often taken for walks in my pushchair.

When we had thunderstorms, which seemed to be more frequent than they are today, my mother insisted that we all gathered in the downstairs back room, close to the dividing wall with the next-door house. In this location, she believed we would be safe if the house collapsed. So, regardless of the time of day - or night for that matter - this was where we huddled. I think she associated thunderstorms with the zeppelin raids of the First World War. She had this fear to the end of her long life.

Next door to us lived a member of the Westminster Church Choir, Mr William Henry Bullock, who sang bass. After a probation period he was promoted to lay vicar in 1912. He continued with the choir until his retirement in 1935.

It was during our time in this house that my mother insisted that I had elocution lessons, so that I 'talked proper', and during the summer months there were gatherings in our garden when our class had to perform before family and friends. I expect there was also a collection for a charity, probably the League of Pity, the junior branch of the National Society for the Prevention of Cruelty to Children (NSPCC).

Until I started school (after that it could only be during school holidays), my mother and I made bus trips to Kensington High Street so that she could look around the large stores - *Barkers, Deny & Toms*, and *Pontings*. She would have a cup of tea in the roof garden restaurant of *Deny & Toms* where a small orchestra would be playing - a friend of hers was the violinist. The fare was 4d and I travelled free until I was age three when it went up to half fare.

There were no automatic lifts or escalators in those days and every lift had an attendant who opened and closed the lift gates. They then pulled a rope up or down according to the direction of travel - great fun but rather frightening to a small boy. If my mother wanted something special, or Auntie Stella had written from India asking her to obtain some special dress material for herself or her children, we would travel to Oxford Street (7d fare), have a budget lunch at *Bourne & Hollingsworth*, and then walk along Oxford Street looking in the shop windows. I wasn't aware in those days that *Hamleys* toy store was only a short distance down Regent Street from Oxford Circus. If only I had known!

Being so near to central London, we also attended an evening performance of a pantomime at a West End theatre each year - very lavish productions in those days. We travelled back on the upper deck of the bus so that we could see the ever changing coloured lights at Piccadilly Circus advertising *Bovril* and other products. I also enjoyed two annual events at Olympia. The first was the Royal Tournament (a display by the three services of the armed forces in aid of their charities), the second, the Ideal Home Exhibition. We went as a family to the former, my father being particularly

46

interested in the gun carrier event by the Royal Horse Artillery - he was attached to this regiment when he was in the Territorial Army before the First World War. My mother and I attended the latter and I always came home with a supply of the miniature pots of preserves.

Visits to my grandparents at Erith, Kent, were quite an adventure for a small boy, especially before the track from London to Erith was electrified. The first part of the journey was on an electric train along the Mortlake to Waterloo line. After walking over to Waterloo Junction (not Waterloo East in those days), we then climbed aboard a steam hauled train bound for Erith (about a 20-minute journey). The final part of the journey was by tram from Erith Station up the hill to Northumberland Heath. In those days the trams terminated here and if you wanted to travel on to Bexleyheath, you had to change to a different type of tram.

We would usually have lunch with Granny Mohr, visit my father's parents (only five minutes walk away) in the afternoon, and travel home after tea. It was a much greater adventure in winter, especially if it was foggy for the return journey. If my mother and I made the journey during the week, when my father was at work, it was less costly to have a cheap day ticket from Mortlake to Vauxhall. From here, a London County Council tram would take us to Abbey Wood terminus where we would change to the Erith tram. Although this was a cheaper way to travel, it was much slower.

Most trains in those days had a display board below the luggage rack. On these were posted pictures of places of interest that could be visited by trains of the region (i.e. *Great Western, London Midland & Scottish, London & North Eastern, Southern*). The boards were also used for advertising. One such poster on our electric service to Waterloo was for *Hovis*. It showed a picture of the front of five *Southern Electric* trains with five different head codes - viz. H, O, V, I, S - with the information that 'H' destination from Waterloo was Hampton Court (later when the line to Guildford via Effingham Junction was electrified a bar on top indicated destination Guildford); 'O' was Kingston via Richmond; 'V' was Kingston via Wimbledon; 'I' was Isleworth and 'S', Shepperton. When more lines were electrified, especially on the south eastern section from London Bridge, numbers instead of letters were used for these codes.

47

Once or twice a year we would spend the weekend with my cousins at Bush Hill Park, north London. Travel would be by bus to Hammersmith Broadway, then Piccadilly line underground train to Finsbury Park (the full length of the line in those days). A tram then took us to Wood Green, where we changed to a bus *en route* to Bush Hill Park. Before new train stock with automatic doors was installed on the Piccadilly Line in the mid-20s, every carriage had an open platform at either end with a guard who would open and close the metal gates at each station. Once the gates were secured, he would give a bell signal to the guard on the next rear carriage. This guard would in turn ring his bell, and so on, until the signal reached the guard in the last carriage. This final guard had the job of waving his green flag to the driver to indicate that the train could depart. These were very noisy trains and there was much screeching of wheels on bends. Similar stock was still being used on the Waterloo to Bank line, known as 'The Sewer', at the outbreak of World War II.

From my earliest days to the outbreak of the Second World War, we spent every Christmas at Leytonstone, East London, with the Gill family - Auntie Alice, Uncle Horace, Nell, Mary, Con, the twins, and Bill (who was 16 months older than me). Offices did not close on Christmas Eve as they do today, so my father went to work that day, meeting my mother and me at Bank mid-afternoon. We then travelled together either on a very slow, dirty steam train from Liverpool Street (the *Central Line* extension was not opened until after World War II) or by bus or tram from Aldgate to Leytonstone station. The final stretch to Wallwood Road was on foot.

* * * * *

The holiday tended to follow a set pattern - bridge for the adults and billiards (Uncle Horace had a full-size table in his basement) for the men. There were no freezers in those days and so everyone had to purchase their turkey as near to Christmas Day as possible. The cheapest turkeys were to be found in the markets and these could be bought at bargain prices on Christmas Eve, the vendors not wishing to store them over the Christmas holiday. The later in the day the purchase was made, the cheaper the turkeys became and, much to everyone's concern, Uncle Horace would visit a London market as late as possible on Christmas Eve to purchase his 'bird'. On Christmas morning he would take on the responsibility of cooking it in the large, old gas oven (only used at Christmas) conveniently situated near the billiard room. From this position he could enjoy his game whilst basting the bird at the same time. The rest of the family had to slave away in the kitchen above!

Sometimes the younger children, including me, would be sent out for a walk on Wanstead Flats. It could be bitterly cold and our fingers and toes became so chilled that I often cried bitterly when we arrived back at the house.

At lunchtime on Christmas Day, we would be joined by Uncle Lawrence (Uncle Horace's brother) and his large family. They generally stayed on for the afternoon and then, after tea, we usually trooped a few houses up the road to sing carols with another part of the family. I suspect this involved another game of billiards and a drink. This house also had Christmas guests, the Wootton's, another part of the family who, at that time, lived in Southampton. They included my cousin Dick.

IT was a ten minute walk to Uncle Lawrence's house where, on Boxing Day, we had lunch with his family, and generally stayed there until after midnight. Everybody looked forward to this Boxing Day meal there were newly-minted coins in the Christmas pudding, courtesy of Uncle Lawrence who was employed at the Bank of England. After supper there was always the traditional dancing of the *Roger de Coverley*, in which everyone participated, and sometimes a family pantomime. We are still in touch with one of Uncle Lawrence's grandchildren, Margaret, the daughter of the late Donald and Marjorie Gill. Margaret now lives near Hereford.

* * * * *

The population of Great Britain was obviously greatly affected by The Great War, as World War I was then known, and my mother was no exception. She had soldiers of a Scottish regiment billeted with her when my father was serving with the RNAS. Some were killed on the battlefield shortly after leaving her for France and I am quite sure that she corresponded not only with their colleagues, but also with their parents. Many relatives of her friends were also killed in action. When peace was declared, my mother and father joined with the cheering crowds in central London.

Armistice Day, when the fallen are remembered, was always on November 11th, irrespective of the day of the week (it was not until after the Second World War that it was changed to Remembrance Sunday). For several years everybody and everything remaining silent for two minutes at 11am; all traffic came to a halt and many of the trains also stopped wherever they were, even if between stations. Maroons set off at every police station signalled the beginning and end of the two minute period. Mother and I often travelled up to London to join the crowd around the Cenotaph in Whitehall. One year we stayed at home in East Sheen to attend the unveiling of the new war memorial in Sheen Lane.

One of the highlights of living in East Sheen was the annual Oxford and Cambridge intervarsity boat race, rowed each year from Putney to Mortlake. For a fortnight or more before the race many of the shops had dark blue and light blue favours for sale (for a price of 1d upwards), and it seemed that everyone was wearing one on the day of the race. Ratepayers were able to obtain special spectator places in the council's boatyard. Sometimes, through the kindness of friends of the family, we were able to view the race from one of the brewery's windows overlooking the river. It was always a great day out and a most memorable occasion - no TV in those days! I supported Cambridge, for the simple reason that they were the crew that won the race the first year that I watched it.

* * * * *

Summer holidays were something I greatly looked forward to. The journey was probably more exciting than nowadays when so much travelling is by car. The main luggage was sent 'luggage in advance' (cost one shilling). It was collected by the railway carrier on the Friday morning and would be at our destination when we arrived on the Saturday afternoon. We went to Torquay one year and I can remember the fishmonger touring the streets in the early morning shouting, "Mackerel! Fresh mackerel!"

For several years after that, our fortnight summer holiday was spent at Croyde Bay, North Devon, which in those days was a very quiet seaside resort with no hotels and rarely more than three families sharing the vast expanse of sands. The horse-drawn hansom cab from Mortlake station would transport us from home to the station, from whence we travelled by electric train to Waterloo. At Waterloo we would transfer to the Ilfracombe section of the *Atlantic Coast Express*. On alighting at Braunton, a taxi would take us to Croyde. The long journey was broken by having lunch in the restaurant car on the train; one of the highlights of the day.

The *Atlantic Coast Express* conveyed carriages for various destinations, including South Devon coastal resorts, Bude and Bideford on the north coast; these were detached from the train at the appropriate junction and pulled to their various destinations by local engines. On the return journey to London, these coaches would be waiting at the junction to be reattached to the main train.

When I was older and at my first school, I made the journey to Croyde alone, travelling in the guard's van in the care of the guard. It was during the Easter holidays and I stayed with one of my mother's friends. In a similar manner I once travelled to Bath where Auntie Stella was living on one of her furloughs from India. On this train we travelled in a 'slip coach', which the guard operated as we approached Bath station - very exciting. On another occasion I, together with my bicycle, travelled from Euston to Birmingham New Street station to visit my mother's aunt, Auntie Florrie, who lived at 27 Wilton Road, Sparkhill. I remember taking all my *Meccano* with me.

After I started school, we had two holidays abroad. The first was at Heyst-sur-mer in Belguim, from where we enjoyed several day tours by charabanc around the First World War battlefields. From here we also visited Bruge, and crossed the border into Holland where we had a ride on the steam tram from Knocke. The second holiday was to Jersey in the Channel Islands. Air travel was not common in those days and these holidays involved travel by sea. We sailed from Dover for our Belgian holiday and Weymouth for our trip to the Channel Islands. In Weymouth, the boat train was pulled by a tank engine through the streets of the town to the dockside.

Other family holidays, before I started camping, were to Newquay, Cornwall, and Sandown, Isle of Wight; on the latter, my mother was able to play tennis and there were paddle boats at the recreation ground for me. I can also remember spending a few days during one of the school Easter holidays at Selsey, Sussex - this entailed travelling from Victoria to Chichester by main line steam train and then on a narrow gauge steam railway for the remainder of the journey.

It must have been shortly after we moved to Palwell Park that my mother joined an arts and crafts club in Richmond. She also joined a mandolin band. The former introduced her to pokerwork and all her friends and family will remember the pokerwork gifts they received at Christmas. We still have some of her larger creations in our home today. The leader of the mandolin band was Doris Lancaster, a music teacher in Richmond. Unfortunately, she was forced to move away (on the advice of her doctors after she developed TB) and ended up living in Croyde. Despite the loss of its leader, the band met regularly in members' houses during the winter months, often having a combined music and bridge evening. This interest in music, and the fact that it was the done thing for a child to learn a musical instrument, resulted in my having to have piano lessons, and later violin lessons - I never enjoyed these.

Another of my mother's hobbies was photography. She started with a *Box Brownie* and later bought a more sophisticated camera. With the help of my father, and using the cupboard under the stairs as a dark room, she undertook her own developing and printing.

These were the days when Saturday mornings were part of the working week. On his way home from his business office in the City, my father would purchase a box of *Fullers* peppermint creams for my mother, and sometimes a bottle of barley sugar for me.

How technology has moved on since my childhood days. I can just remember my father bringing home one of the first wireless sets. He may have purchased it at *Gamages* in Holborn, but I rather suspect that it came from one of his city friends who was an amateur enthusiast. You had to adjust a 'whisker' onto a rod to receive a signal from the broadcasting station (Savoy Hill) and then listen to the rather crackling sound through earphones; my interest was *Children's Hour*, with the various aunts and uncles and their birthday messages.

Later we had a set with liquid low tension batteries (accumulators), which had to be charged regularly at a local shop (you had to be careful not to spill the acid liquid), and a large, heavy, high tension battery. The latter was eventually replaced by a transformer that you plugged into the house electricity supply. The sets had several large valves that needed replacing from time to time and there was a separate loudspeaker. In these early days there was only one broadcasting station in the London area (2LO) and, except for special sporting occasions (e.g. test matches, Wimbledon tennis championship), programmes did not commence until early evening. It was many years before more modern sets with internal speakers were marketed.

* * * * *

Whilst we were living in East Sheen, a great friend of mine was a boy called Warwick. He lived in a large house at the bottom of Richmond Park Road with his parents, his younger brother Michael, and an aunt (his mother's sister, I think). Warwick's father was one of the treasurers of Mortlake parish church. We spent much time at each other's houses, playing with our toys and inventing new games. We enjoyed putting on shows, particularly after one of us had been given an amateur conjuring set for Christmas, and we learnt to perform various tricks. We had our own secret codes too but, much to our dismay, Warwick's aunt, having been in the Secret Service during the First World War, was able to decipher them easily! Our friendship dwindled after we started to attend different schools and when my parents and I moved to Hinchley Wood, I ceased to hear much about him. However, my mother did keep in touch with his mother for many years and I understand that his outlook on life was much affected by his wartime experiences, which included being evacuated from Dunkirk.

A few years after the end of the First World War, following the sale of part of the extensive grounds of Sheen House in Sheen Lane (the home and surgery of Dr Hovenden), a new estate was developed. Between the existing Sheen Lane and Richmond Park Road, a new road, named Shrewsbury Avenue, was constructed. This resulted in the creation of a triangular piece of land bordered by existing houses in Sheen Lane and new homes being built in Richmond Park Road and Shrewsbury Avenue. On this piece of land a tennis club was developed. It consisted of five hard court tennis courts, two lawns for miniature golf, and a pavilion with separate changing rooms and toilets for ladies and gentlemen. There was a balcony connecting these, off which was the Club House with a kitchen at the rear that was used for serving teas at weekends and soft drinks when needed. There were two table-tennis tables, and the room was also used for club meetings and various other activities. There was no licensed bar.

The old Sheen House stables, on the corner of Sheen Lane and Shrewsbury Avenue, were purchased by a veterinary surgeon who developed them to provide stabling for the horses of those who rode in Richmond Park. He also ran a clinic and offered boarding facilities for small domestic animals - this is where Mick stayed when we went on holiday.

This new tennis club was registered as a limited company and each person joining the club purchased shares to help finance the project. The board of directors included Dr Hovenden, Mr Watts (no relation to my father's boss in the City) who, like my father, purchased a house in Richmond Park Road, and Mr Woolridge who lived in one of the houses in Sheen Lane backing on to the club. My father was the non-salaried company secretary. A groundsman, Mr Ford, was appointed to tend the tennis courts and generally care for the grounds and pavilion.

The club was open every day of the week except Sunday mornings, Good Friday, and certain days around Christmas, and our lives very much evolved around it. My mother was one of best underhand tennis servers in the locality. She entered all the annual tournaments and the bank holiday knock-out tournaments held at the club, and also played in matches against other clubs. Over the years she won many prizes. She was a regular attendee at the Lawn Tennis Championships at Wimbledon, but only as a spectator!

The cigarettes for sale at the club were delivered to our house and kept in a drawer of the dressing table in our spare bedroom. Every Friday in the summer, a van from *Jo Lyons* would deliver fruit cakes, chocolate cup cakes, jam sandwiches, and the like, for sale by Mr Ford at the weekend.

The club grounds provided an excellent playground for us youngsters on our 'fairy' bikes, but our parents forbade our riding there on busy summer weekends. The club also organised various coach outings. I remember going to the military tattoos at Wembley during the 1924 and 1925 Empire Exhibitions, and later the tattoos at Aldershot.

Most roads were not busy with traffic in those days. I was free to ride my bike on the pavement wherever I liked, providing I did not cross the Upper Richmond Road which was one of the main thoroughfares from central London to Richmond and beyond. I was able to go shopping for my mother to *Montagues* (the greengrocers), *Ashton's* (the ironmongers), *Peck's* (the haberdashers) and other shops on our side of this main road. A butcher from Mortlake used to call for our weekend joint order on Friday morning for delivery on Saturday morning. The milkman would deliver twice daily, early morning and again mid-morning, and the baker would call every day. There were three postal deliveries every day and a letter posted in central London before midday would be delivered the same day! The street lamps were lit by gas. The lamp lighter was very agile with his rod and did not alight from his bicycle to light the lamps.

Each morning my father purchased the *Daily Telegraph* to read on the train on his way to work. We also had two tabloid newspapers, the *Daily Mirror* and *Daily Sketch* - the children's section of the former had the Pip, Squeak, and Wilfred Club whilst the latter ran the Gug Nunk Club. I was also a member of the junior section of the NSPCC (the League of Pity) and helped at fêtes, etc.

When we moved to Richmond Park Road, a very pleasant Sunday routine gradually developed. Early in the morning, before the rest of the household were awake, I would set off on my fairy bike, accompanied by our dog Mick, and cycle through Richmond Park from Sheen Gate to Roehampton Gate. In these days no cars were allowed in the park (except special traffic to White Lodge), the roads being restricted to horse riders and horse-drawn vehicles. We would then proceed along Roehampton Lane, Priory Lane, and into the Upper Richmond Road, continuing along this road as far as the junction with Richmond Park Road. From here we headed home. Once home, I would cook sausages, our Sunday morning treat.

Mid-morning, my father and I would set off walking through the park from Sheen Gate to Richmond Gate. From here we went down through the gardens to the towpath of the River Thames, then home by bus. Our route took us past the Nissen huts that used to be occupied by soldiers of World War I, and were still situated in the park close to Richmond Gate. Just outside was the newly built Star & Garter Home for disabled ex-servicemen. Situated in the valley below was the British Legion poppy factory which produced all the poppies for sale each November. In those days these were all made by hand by ex-service personnel.

In the summer, as an alternative, we might take the number 33 bus to Hampton Court, passing through Twickenham and Bushy Park, returning on a number 73 via Kingston-upon-Thames and Ham. A variation of this was to catch a bus to Richmond, take the Messrs. Mears paddle steamer to Hampton Court (passing through Teddington Lock and Kingston-upon-Thames), and return home by bus.

In the afternoon, Mother and I would attend the children's service at Christ Church, located close to Sheen Common. The church was built in 1864, with a donation from Queen Victoria, to serve the expanding population of this part of the parish. As a treat for me, particularly on such days as Easter, Harvest Festival and Remembrance Sunday, we would all attend the evening service at Mortlake parish church.

As the population grew, it was decided that a third church was needed and All Saints was built at the top of East Sheen Avenue. The foundation stone was laid in October 1928 by the Duchess of York, whose home at that time was in the parish at White Lodge, Richmond Park.

It was when we were living in East Sheen that our first telephone was connected. There were no automatic dialling telephones in those days; all calls were connected by the operator.

My main hobbies were *Meccano* and a gauge 0 *Hornby* model railway - the smaller 00 gauge was a much later development. I used to create large models with the *Meccano* - ships, lifts, cranes - and, when I had a motor for it, various lorries and cars. It was great fun and, as well as being educational, kept me occupied for hours. In earlier years I also had a model farm. I bought the various animals and farm equipment from either the Post Office stores or the toyshop in Sheen Lane.

I think that my father brought my first train set home with him following a business trip to Germany - it was a *Bing*, a rather tinny clockwork model with a simple oval track. I obviously had this set before September 1923, as there is a letter of this date from my maternal great grandfather saying, 'I am sending you a little present to let you know that I have not forgotten your last birthday. It is a little station where your trains can run to.'

One Christmas I was given my first *Hornby* clockwork tank engine train set. Presents in subsequent years included a main line *London, Midland and Scottish* engine, *Pullman* cars, goods trucks and many other accessories, such as points and crossovers. Over the years this gradually developed into quite a large track which extended from my bedroom in the front of the house, along the upstairs landing, and into and around the spare back bedroom. The only problem was that I had to dismantle it every evening before going to bed!

When we later moved to Hinchley Wood, the track was laid in the loft and electrified using a third central rail. In this permanent location we were soon able to develop it further. At Hinchley Wood I also attempted to build an outside track, laying it on shelves attached to the fence, with the terminus in the tool shed. Despite the fact that we used non-rust track, it was never really satisfactory. Atmospheric conditions soon affected the track, resulting in poor electrical contact between track and engine.

When we moved from Hinchley Wood in 1939, I reluctantly dismantled the track and packed it away. My model railway ambitions had to be put on hold until Jonathan was a few years old and we were living in Bromsgrove. Here we built an 00 gauge track all around his bedroom.

The first school I attended, from September 1925, was the mixed kindergarten class at the County School for Girls, Parkshot, Richmond (I think I attended a small Montessori school in Sheen Lane before this, for a few mornings each week). The school was situated close to Richmond station and my mother was able to take me every day for the first few months. I then went with an older girl who lived opposite us in Richmond Park Road and was also a pupil. I have copies of the papers that my father signed before I was admitted - the fees were £4.00 per term (plus ten shillings for books), and 10d per day for school lunch.

Although the school was founded in 1861 as a 'ladies establishment for gentlemen's daughters', the main buildings were quite new, the school having been rebuilt in 1909 at a cost of £19,252 14s. 8d! Pupil numbers increased so greatly following the construction of the new housing developments in the neighbourhood that in 1920, a line of wooden huts, jettisoned after the First World War, were erected in the very extensive grounds. The headmistress was Miss E.M. Weeks and one of my teachers was called Miss Stratton. I can remember little of my time at the school except the nature walks in Old Deer Park and that we had a bun and a glass of milk at mid-morning break at the cost of 1d. It was great fun getting to and from school during the general strike of 1926 - we just walked down to the Upper Richmond Road and travelled on whatever transport came along, whether it be a bus, private car, or even a lorry! We usually arrived at school on time, but everyone realised the situation and were glad to see us whatever time we arrived.

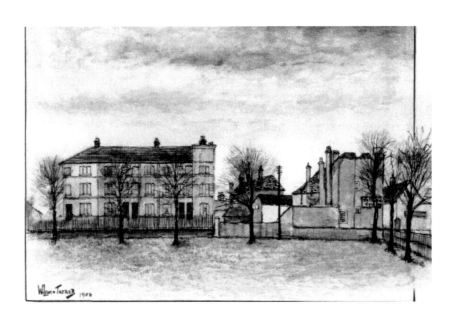

Cromwell Place, Mortlake, where I was born

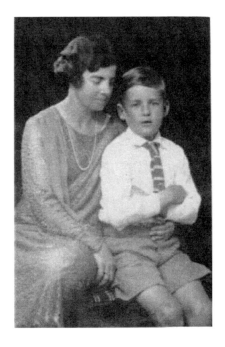

With my mother

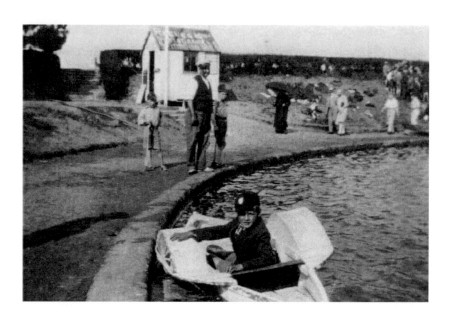

On holiday in Sandown, Isle of Wight c1925

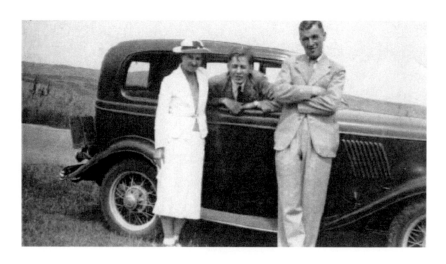

Our first car, registration PJ 9771, c1937

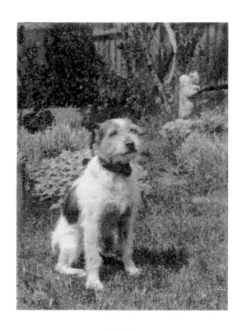

Mick

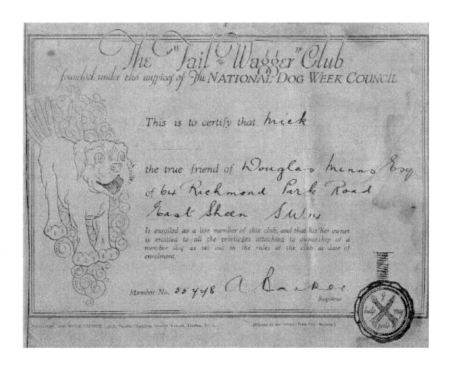

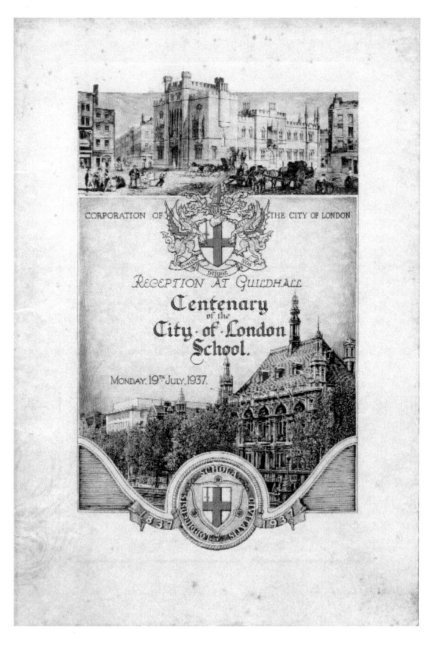

Cover of City of London School Centenary Brochure
Top: The original School in Milk Lane
Bottom: The Victoria Embankment building

Carpenter's Children

I entered the City of London School (CLS) in January 1929. Although there was no entrance examination in those days, you did have to be recommended by one of the City Aldermen. I was taken to meet one of these gentlemen in his office. He more or less just shook hands with me and wished me well at the school. Then, the term before I commenced at the school, I had to attend an appointment with the headmaster, the Rev Dr Arthur Chilton. My 'test' was to read a passage from a book and answer a few mathematical questions. Having clearly performed to his satisfaction, I became one of 'Carpenter's Children'. Let me explain.

The founder of CLS was John Carpenter, a town clerk and also a friend of Sir Richard (Dick) Whittington. (Dick Whittington was not just a legend from a fairy story, but a real man, and it is a historical fact that he was four times Lord Mayor of London in the 14th and 15th centuries.) On his death in 1442, John Carpenter left £16.11s for the education of four poor boys, to be called Carpenter's Children. By 1834 there was enough money to open a school for 200 boys, not quite so poor, but still surprisingly unpretentious by the standards of the time. The first building was in Honey Lane Market, Cheapside, and it was opened in 1837. By 1883, a purpose built school had been constructed on the Victoria Embankment on the edge of the city boundary, the opening ceremony being performed by the Prince of Wales (later King Edward VII). With further extension it could, by the time I became a pupil, accommodate over 700 pupils. There was now also a City of London School for girls on the other side of Sion College.

I started at the bottom of the school in the class known as the 3rd junior, with 'Daddy' Grover as our form master; except for gym lessons, I think that he was the only person to teach us during these first two terms at the school. I was in Mortimer House, named after a one time headmaster of the school. The first day was not a very happy one, mainly because my parents had misread the dress instructions and timetables. Every boy was supposed to wear a suit, but I was dressed in short trousers and a sweater. The next day my mother met me after school (it was a Wednesday - the school half-day). We lunched at *Unilever House* then went to *Swan & Edgar*, Piccadilly Circus, the official school outfitters, and bought me a new suit - short trousers and a jacket.

The second dilemma, involving the timetable, resulted in me having to wait three-quarters of an hour for my father. He had told me to meet him outside the school at 3.30pm (the normal finishing time for all other forms), but afternoon school for the 3rd junior actually ended at 2.45pm. When he finally arrived, he took me on the bus to Waterloo station where he saw me safely onto the train from which my mother met me at Mortlake station.

My father met me like this (during his extended tea-break) fairly regularly for several terms, often buying me a bag of cherries or a peach from the station fruit stall. After this, I used to travel all the way on my own. I remember walking up Sheen Lane from the station looking in the toyshops. I especially liked the one selling *Meccano*. The policeman on point duty saw me safely across the busy Upper Richmond Road at Perrings Corner; this was long before traffic lights were installed.

In the mornings, I travelled on the same commuter train to Waterloo as my father, and we then took a number 76 bus along Stamford Street and over Blackfriars Bridge. I alighted at Blackfriars whilst my father continued on the bus to Bank. The train line between Mortlake and Waterloo ran close to the Thames and it could be very foggy in the winter - real 'pea soupers'. Hence, progress could be very slow - semaphore signalling was still in operation and with no coloured light sections, the driver had to depend on fog men in their little huts by the side of the line activating maroon-type warning devices. We could be very late for school on such days, but so too were many of the masters!

During my second year at the school, the lower forms were invited to a demonstration of the newest craze, the Yo-Yo. It was not long before all the boys had one or more of these 'scientific' toys but they were soon banned for use within the school buildings and only allowed in the playground.

Occasionally a guest lecturer was invited to the school, usually at the end of afternoon lessons, and pupils of the appropriate age group were invited to attend. These lectures were held in the upper lecture theatre which was right at the top of the building, accessed via a narrow staircase from the third floor. In the lecture theatre was one of the old-type magic lanterns using 3-inch square glass slides. Illumination was provided by electricity being passed through two carbon electrodes, which resulted in a bright light. The lectures were great fun and usually educational!

Once or twice a year, on a Wednesday afternoon, there were optional educational trips to such places within the London area as *Fords* at Dagenham, a cold storage depot at a nearby Thames wharf, a sweet factory, a telephone exchange, and other such commercial establishments.

One of the disadvantages of being at school in a different area from where one lived (pupils attended from all over London and its suburbs), was that most of one's school friends lived quite a distance away from you. One of my friends was Merideth Budd. He joined the school at the same time as myself and lived in Earls Court. To visit him from home I had to travel by bus to Kensington cinema where he would meet me and take me back to his flat. His bedroom, in which he had a model railway on shelves around the wall, overlooked the *District Line* railway junction to the west of Earls Court station where lines to Olympia and Wimbledon branched from the main line. This was of great interest to me. Budd became a Company Sergeant Major in the school OTC and when war was declared, trained as an army officer. He reached the rank of Major and made the army his career, serving most of his time in the Middle East. I never met him again after we left school but we regularly exchanged Christmas cards. Budd never married and on retirement lived in Andalucia.

In September 1931, my cousin Bill Gill joined the school. Bill was 15 months older than me and stayed at the school until he sat his school certificate examination in July 1935. Most Saturday mornings we met at Waterloo station and travelled together to the school sports ground at Grove Park, Kent, for athletics, cricket or rugger, depending on the season of the year. Bill joined the school rowing club when it was formed in 1934 and became their cox. Our parents often attended the annual sports day held just before Easter. I was never very good at sport and was never a member of any house or school teams. Towards the end of my time at the school I did represent them at chess, visiting polytechnics and other schools around London for matches. We once played against Ramsgate School.

I was also a member of the newly formed school choir. The older boys sang tenor or bass whilst the Temple and Chapel Royal choristers, who received free education at CLS, sang the other parts. We sang at the Guildhall School of Music before the school dramatic society productions, and also at an official reception at the Guildhall held to mark the centenary of the school.

Bill sometimes stayed with me during the holidays and we used to cycle from Hinchley Wood to Ashford (Middlesex) to visit our cousin Dick Wootton. The only problem was that Dick lived next door to our senior chemistry master who had a large greenhouse which did not take kindly to cricket balls!

The schoolday started with us all gathering in the Great Hall at 9.05 am for morning prayers - never called 'assembly' in those days. These was taken by the headmaster who, after any notices (following which those of the Jewish faith left the hall), led the school in the collect for the day, the school prayer, the Lord's prayer and other appropriate prayers. We would then proceed in silence to our respective classes. If the headmaster was absent for any reason, then the second master, Mr Nobbs, took his place and read the prayers in record time!

Our break for lunch lasted only 35 minutes, with the vast majority of boys and staff having a cooked lunch in *Roach's* at one shilling a day - Roach was the appointed caterer for the Corporation of London. This was a very substantial meal, with choices for both courses, and much appreciated by the majority.

Dr Chilton retired as headmaster in the summer of 1929 and Mr F.R. Dale was appointed his replacement. I am told that he introduced many changes to the curriculum and was quite often seen walking around the school and visiting class lessons. Within a year of taking up his appointment, he brought regularity to the school uniform - black jacket, waistcoat and striped trousers. For those not old enough to wear the seniors' uniform, the dress code was blue serge suit with shorts. No longer was there the variety of attire that had been evident in the past and I am sure that this uniformity helped with the discipline of the school. Teaching staff just had to wear dark suits, but their gowns covered most of these. On speech days they wore their academic hoods which gave a vivid touch of colour to the proceedings - I think those teaching French and Spanish had the brightest ones.

My passage up the school was uneventful. I spent two terms in 3rd Junior, half a term in 2nd Junior, and then the remainder of that year in 1st Junior. This was followed by a year in both Old Grammar and Classical 2a. As well as being taught the usual English, maths, French, etc., we took Latin for most of the time and also one year of Greek. At this level in the school we were divided into sets for maths - I was in the second set for half a term and then promoted to the first set. This meant that we could sit the additional subjects of advanced maths and trigonometry for the School Certificate examinations.

During this period, Unilever House, situated between the school and Blackfriars station, was rebuilt, the noise causing much interruption to lessons. Being on the bank of the Thames, huge steel piles had to be driven a considerable depth into the ground. This was done by very noisy steam pile-drivers. The building was constructed on a steel frame and it was a great sight to watch the red hot rivets, heated at ground level, being thrown to a higher level where they were caught in a gadget held by a workman who then threw them to the next level.

By this time in my schooling, I had already decided that I wanted to become a Dental Surgeon, so my father was advised that I should proceed up the science side of the school. My next form then, was Science 3. I followed this year with a year each in Science 4 and 5, then two years in Science 6, sitting my school certificate in Science 5 and my higher school certificate in Science 6. These were Oxford & Cambridge Joint Board qualifications, of which a combination of the ordinary and higher level certificates fulfilled the requirements for University of London Matriculation. This, in turn, was a necessary requirement for entry to the dental school of the University of London.

During our first year in the sixth, we had our introduction to using public libraries for research, our biology master having carefully removed all reference books for our dissertation on spiders from the school science library! So, on the Saturday morning I had to visit the Surrey County Council Library at Esher and, with the help of the librarian, borrowed any books that they had on this subject. I obtained further books from the headquarter library.

* * * * *

It was shortly after commencing at CLS that I was introduced to Crusaders. One of the boys, Geoffrey Dowse, who was a year ahead of me but travelled on the same train as me to Waterloo, invited me to go along with him to the East Sheen class one Sunday afternoon - I later learnt that they were having a recruiting campaign and his team would gain ten extra points if a member introduced a new recruit! Although Geoffrey moved from the area soon after this, I continued attending and have been a Crusader ever since, moving to different classes according to my place of residence. I eventually became a leader and helped with various Union activities.

I think my mother was a little saddened at first that I had left the church Sunday school but did not influence me in any way and took it all in her stride. I don't think that the class leaders took too kindly to my continuing to attend services at our local Anglican church and tried to influence me to join a local 'evangelical' church by inviting me to attend their evening service with them - they did not succeed.

The sad part was that in those days Crusaders was limited to pupils of public and preparatory schools and, as my friend Warwick attended the local county school, he could not became a member - with the problems he experienced during his wartime service in the army and after demobilisation, it could have made all the difference to him. This situation did change, partly because of changes in the education system, but also as a result of the Christian fellowship that developed in the forces during the Second World War.

I can remember taking part in Crusader sports days at Herne Hill and going on several of the famous Crusader excursions during the Easter holidays. These included the railway works at Swindon and Crewe, the docks at Southampton with a cruise in the Solent, and other educational trips. I never attended a Crusader camp but in 1931 our cousin, Dick Wootton, invited Bill and I to attend a Varsity and Public Schools house party (VPS was part of the Scripture Union movement) at Great Walstead School, Haywards Heath, and for the next three years, the North Wales VPS camp at Fairbourse, Merionethshire (fees were £5.00 for three weeks, which my father could just afford). The camp was largely supported by boys from Highgate School and CLS, with officers from Oxford and Cambridge universities. It is of interest to note that amongst the list of items for camp was a suit for 'travelling and to wear on Sundays'.

The main party travelled to North Wales on the *Cambrian Coast Express* from Paddington via Birmingham (where the railwaymen used to walk down the line tapping all the carriage wheels to make sure none were cracked) and Shrewsbury. There were two sections to the train with a restaurant car in the middle. On reaching Shrewsbury, the train divided, the front section proceeding via Llangollan and Dolgelly to Barmouth and Phewlli (we alighted at Barmouth Junction) and the rear portion going to Aberystwyth via Welshpool and Mahynlyth. One year our reserved coach was on the wrong side of the restaurant car and we had to travel all the way to Mahynlyth. Here we were unhitched and another engine towed us all the way along the coastal line to Barmouth Junction. There was a swing bridge over the estuary between Barmouth Junction and Barmouth and it is here that the film of *The Ghost Train* was filmed.

It was during my second camp in Wales that my mother and father came down to Barmouth for a few days holiday and gave me the sad news that our dog, Mick, had died; we think he had been given poisoned meat by burglars who broke into our house a few months earlier. We could not live without a dog and it was not long before Taffy, a welsh terrier, joined the family. He also joined the Tailwaggers Club.

Between the two world wars, the large rallies for all who had attended Children's Special Service Mission (CSSM) beach summer missions, VPS camps, caravan missions to village children, or were members of the SU, were held each September and January in the Central Hall, Westminster. The young people and their leaders filled the auditorium and then met in their various groups in the basement afterwards for tea. These were great inspirational gatherings for us young people living in such troubled times.

In 1936, Edwin Haigh, a fellow pupil and North Wales camper who lived in Finchley and whose home I had visited on several occasions, suggested that, for a change, we should attend the summer Pioneer camp at Bembridge, Isle of Wight. I knew nothing about the Pioneers but later learnt that they were the home youth group, supporting the South Africa General Mission (which later became the Africa Evangelical Fellowship). David Tryon, a friend of Edwin's, was one of their youth leaders and the commandant of this camp. Thus began a long association with David Tryon and Pioneer camps - I attended four camps (two at Bembridge and two at Seaford, Sussex) before the Second World War, several house parties during the war before I joined the Royal Navy, and many camps thereafter. Although the nature of the camps changed with the times, their biblical content always remained the same. They continued until 2006. I served as a tent officer for several years then, at the 1941 house party at Stamford School, dealt with all the problems associated with rationing. In post-war years, I fulfilled many other staff officer duties.

* * * * *

With many Crusaders at CLS, there was a very active and well attended Christian Union (CU) which met every Tuesday at 3.35 pm in Room 3, the meeting lasting for half an hour. Being situated in the centre of London, we were fortunate in that there were many people working nearby who could be invited as guest speakers and a suitable programme was arranged by our pupils' committee. There were also members of staff, in particular Mr Carey Oakley, who attended whenever they were free - the only time that I can remember the headmaster attending was when Bishop Taylor Smith was our guest! After most meetings, one or two of the senior boys would entertain the speaker to tea (bread, jam, and cakes) in one of the small basement cafés in Bridge Street.

The CU continued right through the war years but in the post-war era, with the large increase in after-school activities and many other factors, attendance numbers diminished and weekly meetings were no longer practicable. The whole nature of Christian witness within the school changed and a new programme to meet modern trends developed. However, there was always an Old Citizens' Prayer Fellowship supporting Christian activities within the school and this is still very active today.

* * * * *

In 1932, gloom struck. It was a Wednesday. I was at home doing my homework and my mother was out on one of her bridge afternoons. My father arrived home at about 3.00 pm instead of his usual 6.30 pm, a most unusual event. He said that he was not unwell and it transpired that his boss, Mr Watts (no family connection with Mr Watts, the father of my friend Bob who lived a few doors up the road), had died a few months earlier - a fact that my mother knew - and those who had taken over the firm had told my father that morning that they no longer required his services. The country was in the grips of the Depression and there was no redundancy pay in those days.

My father remained optimistic but my mother, quite understandably, took the news very badly. He tried to get employment with other firms through his many contacts, but his business friends were either unwilling or unable to help him. As explained in the first chapter, with the help of Uncle Horace he did eventually form his own company - *Munns Gill and Company* - but, despite much hard work, this never really flourished. With war clouds gathering, the Government introduced regulations requiring commercial firms to provide air raid shelters for their employees, and my father did obtain some commissioned work with a firm supplying these shelters but he was without any regular paid employment until he joined the MoS shortly after the outbreak of the war.

My mother used her small savings to buy a second-hand car, a Ford 8 (PJ9771), and, after passing her driving test, was able to drive my father around Surrey on his business trips. My father never learnt to drive himself, although he did undertake maintenance of the car.

Fortunately my father had paid off the mortgage on the house and it was decided that we should sell up and raise a new mortgage on a cheaper property, thereby releasing some capital. Property further out from the centre of London was much cheaper and so we moved to a developing area at Hinchley Wood, between Thames Ditton and Esher, in Surrey, at the end of recently built Kingston-By-Pass.

In actual fact, our new house, although considerably cheaper than the one in East Sheen, was more roomy, was detached, and also had a garage. It was in Manor Road North and we named it *Luxeuil*, after a town in France where my father had been stationed during the First World War. It was very convenient for travelling into London as there was a frequent, fast service from the newly built Hinchley Wood station, non-stop from Surbiton to Waterloo. There was also a half-hourly Green Line coach service along the Kingston-By-Pass to Hammersmith (ls.6d return) and Oxford Circus (2s.3d return).

Another amenity was a tennis club (with bridge as a sideline), of which, as previously mentioned, my mother became a regular member, and also the small Thames Ditton Crusader class for me. Shortly after we moved to Hinchley Wood, an evening badminton club was formed in the newly built Thames Ditton scout hall. This was on a Friday evening and as soon as I was 16, I was able to join (weekend homework could be done on Saturday). My mother was already a member.

We designed our new garden with a concrete-lined pond (no synthetic pond liners in those days) and a rockery. For the latter we used stones dug up from our driveway, which the builders had to realign when the road was completed. We were plagued with moles in the back garden because the land had originally been part of a farmer's field. In my part of the garden I grew vegetables, selling the surplus to neighbours. I used part of the proceeds to purchase seeds for the following year, with any profit left over going to charity.

We purchased our first refrigerator whilst living here. It was operated by gas not electricity.

I have already mentioned my unsuccessful outdoor train track. As I gradually found my way around London, I discovered the *Bassett Lowke* shop near Holborn underground station where they sold track suitable for outside and from where I bought various accessories. I read in 2008 that this company had designed model train layouts on the brand new 115,000-ton *P&O* super liner. I also found various model railway displays, such as in Gamages, High Holborn, only a short walk from the school.

It was around this time that I started to have sickness headaches - I expect they would be called migraines nowadays. When these occurred at school I was taken to the physics laboratory as Mr Pike, the technician, had St John's Ambulance qualifications. Being a day school, there was no sickbay and I had to lie on the floor with a blanket to keep me warm. The headaches usually subsided by the end of the afternoon and I was allowed to travel home by myself on the train. Fortunately, I grew out of these migraines before I left school.

In my O-level year I had suspected appendicitis. The pain was so bad that our local doctor referred me to the Royal Masonic Hospital at Ravenscourt Park, near Hammersmith (my father being a Freemason), and I was an in-patient there for five or six days. No operation was necessary as it turned out and there has been no re-occurrence since then. My only other medical problem was hay fever, from which I suffered each summer for as far back as I can remember. This continued right up to the time I went to sea after I joined the Royal Navy. The chemist at Hinchley Wood suggested some foul tasting medicine but this never did any good - I suspect that it was some herbal remedy!

* * * * *

As a sort of compensation for having to leave my friends behind in East Sheen when we moved to Hinchley Wood, my father gave me a road bike. I was not allowed to ride along the Kingston-By-Pass, or along the main road up to Esher (the roads were too busy), but it was possible, by rather circuitous routes, to ride to the centre of Esher and also around the back of Surbiton and Kingston and then into Richmond Park at the Kingston Gate, leaving by the East Sheen Gate. By now cars were allowed in the park, but with a rigidly enforced 10mph speed limit for cars in the park, riding a bike was quite safe and often quicker!

I also had a Warnford model aircraft at this time and was able to fly it on Telegraph Hill, between Hinchley Wood and Claygate. One had to wind it up with strong elastic and, with careful adjustments of the wings and tail fin, it was possible to keep it in the air for several minutes. On bank holiday Mondays, whilst my mother competed in the tennis club tournaments, my father and I used to walk through Thames Ditton and over Hampton Court bridge to the Fair that was always held on the waste ground opposite Hampton Court palace and gardens. During the school summer holidays I used to pick many pounds of blackberries on Claygate Common so that my mother could make blackberry and apple jam/jelly - I am not sure that she was altogether pleased!

The Thames Ditton Crusader class was a very active one and, as well as the regular Sunday afternoon meetings, the members also played Podex on the village green on Wednesday evenings in the summer, including matches with other nearby classes. Alternative activities were arranged during the winter months.

When I first joined the class, they were meeting in a room over the stable of a large house facing the green. Then the local scouts, having just built their own scout hall, gave Crusaders their old one. I remember it as a rather broken down old wooden ex-army hut, situated between the main Southern Railway line to the south-west and the local line to Claygate and beyond. About a year after we first occupied it, one of the Government departments decided that they needed to widen the road to give better access to their own property, which would necessitate them having to move our hut. We agreed to this, providing they made good any damage to our property, with the result that a previously somewhat dilapidated building became a very acceptable property on good foundation, and it didn't cost the Crusaders a penny - "God moves in a mysterious way ..."

The next step in the renovation of the hut was to improve the interior. One of the leaders of the Kingston class, who owned a timber yard, supplied us with boarding etc. for lining the walls. Gas radiators were also installed and we soon had a warm and cosy building. A large signboard with 'Crusader Hall' written on it was fixed onto the outside of the front of the building and this could be seen by passengers travelling on the main line trains.

Although people were leaving to go to technical college, university or into industry, we retained a very active senior section. We continued as a close-knit community right up to the outbreak of the Second World War.

In the summers of 1937-39 we often cycled to one of the many Surrey villages beyond Leatherhead and Dorking, distributing gospel tracts. I left the district in August 1939 so I do not know what exactly happened to the class except that one of the seniors was killed in action and, after the war, at least three entered the ordained ministry. When I was speaking to one of the members of the National Archives, Kew Friends' Group in the 1990s, I learnt that during in the '60s, the Crusader hut was being used by the young people of St Christopher's Church.

When we first moved to Hinchley Wood, there was no local church, and the vicar from Weston Green held a communion service once a month at the local petrol filling station! It was two years before a Hall Church was built. It was constructed on a site in Upper Claygate Lane, behind where St Christopher's Church was built in the late '50s, when it became their Parish Hall.

This Hall Church served a dual purpose as the Sanctuary could be closed-off with folding doors after any church services and the remainder of the auditorium used for socials, church meetings, badminton, productions of the amateur dramatic society, and various youth groups. I was a Server for a number of years and my mother was in the church choir, as well as being an active in the Mothers' Union. In 1934 I was confirmed in St Paul's Cathedral by the Bishop of London, together with other pupils from the two City of London schools, including my cousin Bill.

Along with other church members, we attended the laying of the foundation stone of the new Guildford Cathedral on Stag Hill, Guildford. There was no problem in parking on the newly constructed Guildford-By-Pass (part of the main route to the important naval town of Portsmouth) as traffic congestion was an unheard of occurrence in those days.

* * * * *

I was 14 in the August after we moved to Hinchley Wood and I had to join the school Officers Training Corps (OTC) at the beginning of the Autumn term. My first taste of army life came the following summer at an OTC camp in the army training area near Strensil, north of York. This qualified me to sit for my 'certificate A' examination the following term, which I passed, and I was promoted to Corporal before the next camp at Bordon, Hampshire. Much to my surprise, I was given the 'Corporals prize' at the OTC concert at the end of the Christmas term following this second camp - the only prize I ever won at the school! The following term I was promoted to Sergeant and had command of my own platoon (number three of 'B' company) during my final year at the school.

The whole corps travelled to either Richmond Park or Wimbledon Common for field days. Those of us who lived in south London could cycle to either Richmond Gate or the top of Wimbledon Hill and join the rest of the Corps there rather than travelling from school by *District Line* train to the nearest station, then marching up to the respective venue. The other annual event was shooting practice on the ranges at Rainham, Essex. There was also a small-bore range opposite the school, under the Victoria Embankment, where we were allowed to practise.

In those days, the OTC also formed part of the Lord Mayors' procession on the 9th November (not necessarily on a Saturday as has been the case since World War II). The procession was not nearly so elaborate as it is nowadays and I usually volunteered to be part of this unit. The one challenge with this was that, in recognition of the great sacrifices made by Old Citizens during World War I, the school OTC had been granted the privilege of marching through the city with fixed bayonets and this made the rifle very heavy on the shoulders. We had watched this event as a family when I was younger, usually from the offices of one of my father's business acquaintances in Queen Victoria Street and, in my early days at the school, from one of the school's front balconies which overlooked the Victoria Embankment.

I can also remember watching the Coronation procession of King George VI and Queen Elizabeth in May 1937, this time from the roof of the Carlton Hotel at the bottom of Haymarket (I think Uncle Bert had been engineer there and my father's firm had supplied them with engineering products in the past). We had a great view as they came along Pall Mall. We did try to make a 9.5mm film of the spectacle but the light was bad and the result very poor. The Corporation of London presented every pupil with a large bar of chocolate in a souvenir box (which I still have to this day) to commemorate the day. We were also given a copy of the official souvenir programme - a very elaborate production with many photographs of the Royal Family, details of the various processions, and an order of service.

Sixth formers at CLS had certain privileges and these I enjoyed for my final two years at the school. We were, for example, allowed to enter the school building by the ornate front door. During morning prayers we stood on the platform facing the rest of the school and during lunch hour we were allowed to stay within the school building rather than being kept outside in the playground, although we did have certain lunch hour duties to perform.

A fellow pupil I remember sitting next to in practical biology lessons was John Stanton. He had spent his earlier school years at Cheefoo School, China (his father being a doctor with the China Inland Mission [CIM], later renamed the Overseas Missionary Fellowship) and, having passed London matriculation, John came to the school to study for higher school certificate subjects before entering medical college. The year was 1935.

A sad event of my last year at CLS was the death of our biology master, Mr WJ.R. Deeks, following a very short illness (polio?) He was a brilliant teacher and was responsible for us obtaining 100% credit pass rate when we sat our school certificate examination. Fortunately, a very energetic supply master filled his place and helped us through our vital examinations.

There were two prize days at the school each year, the main one being in October when the Lord Mayor of London presented the prize. This was quite a formal occasion when, with suitable music being played on the school organ, the Lord Mayor and Sheriffs, preceded by the mace bearer, progressed to the platform. The second was Beaufoy Day in June, this being the occasion when part of a Shakespeare play was performed and special prizes were awarded for performance in English literature examinations at the end of the previous term. A well-known personality in the literature world was the guest of honour on this day. My mother always attended both these occasions.

The other highlight for my mother was the 'Conversazione', held each year just before Christmas and to which all parents of boys in the upper forms were invited. The Lord Mayor and his family always attended and, once all the guests had been received by the headmaster, his wife and members of the school committee, everyone was invited to look around the school and to view various exhibits, including those of a scientific nature by pupils (myself included) from the science forms. I was fortunate in being chosen to demonstrate biology techniques when I had just entered Science 3.

Later there was dancing in the great hall and a cabaret in the gymnasium, more often than not including acts by old boys of the school - the Western Brothers took part one year. Needless to say, there were buffets in various parts of the school and once we had finished our demonstrations, we were able to join in with the festivities, including the many buffets!

My parents attended this event every year and were always very supportive of activities at the school. I can well remember, in my early days at the school, my mother and I attending the funeral in Wimbledon of one of the younger masters, Mr L.G. Sach, who had died after a very short illness (I only knew him because he umpired rugger games at Grove Park). I suspect that my mother had some connection with his mother through the Mothers' Union.

I travelled to and from school every day on the train. During my latter years at the school the track was modernised as part of the electrification of the main line from Waterloo to Portsmouth. This involved the building of a fly-over on the London side of Wimbledon, the development of electric colour light signalling, the modernisation of Surbiton station and, to cope with the ever increasing population in this suburb of London, the building of a new station, Berrylands, between Maldon and Surbiton.

In 1937, the school celebrated its centenary. A Service of Thanksgiving to Almighty God was held at St Paul's Cathedral on Tuesday March 2nd, the sermon being preached by The Very Reverend J.G. Simpson, D.D., a former pupil of the school. During that year there were various other celebratory events, including the whole school being invited by the Lord Mayor to a special afternoon tea at the Mansion House. On Monday 19th July, the Corporation of London gave a reception at the Guildhall to celebrate the occasion. Amongst the entertainment was a recital by the school choir, of which I was a member, with a programme of madrigals and sea shanties. It is also of interest to note that there was a programme of music by the string band of the Honourable Artillery Company, cousin Bill's regiment.

Learning Responsibilities

I left the City of London School in 1937. Unfortunately my higher school certificate passes in chemistry and physics did not qualify me for exemption from the preliminary requirements of the Royal College of Surgeons, as I needed to have studied organic chemistry as well. Consequently, I had to spend a term at Kingston Polytechnic swotting up on this subject and I then took the examination at the end of December. I passed this and secured a place to commence my studies at the Royal Dental Hospital of London, London School of Dental Surgery, in January 1938.

Finance for my course was an issue. There were no government grants in those days and my father could not afford to pay the tuition fees himself. Fortunately, I was awarded a *Times* scholarship from the Corporation of London by my school, and also a bursary from the Dental Board of the United Kingdom (when the National Health Service was introduced in 1948, this Board was disbanded and the General Dental Council established in its place). The application for the bursary was supported by my father's dental surgeon, Doris Thurston (neé Grose), whom I later learnt was the first woman student to qualify from the Royal Dental Hospital (RDH), gaining the Alfred Woodhouse Scholarship during her studies.

The application was followed by an interview with members of the board (a rather harrowing ordeal), some of whom, particularly Mr Ballard (the father of Prof. Cliff Ballard, who became an eminent orthodontist) were very supportive, not only during my student days but throughout my career. I was granted a small initial bursary to enable me to study for my Licentiate in Dental Surgery (LDS) qualification. This was increased some eighteen months later when my father was finding it even more difficult to support me.

Educational grants were another possible source of finance available to me, but because the CLS was situated in the county of Middlesex and we lived in the county of Surrey, neither council would offer me a grant. I was, however, able to obtain a small loan from Surrey. It was fortunate that I, like many other of my fellow students, could live at home and travel to the Dental School each day, thus not having the extra expense of 'digs'..

* * * * *

The history of the evolution of dentistry is an interesting one. In the Medical Act of 1858 (Royal Assent 2nd August) was a clause which read, 'It shall notwithstanding anything herein contained be lawful for Her Majesty by charter, to grant to the Royal College of Surgeons of England power to institute and hold examinations for the purpose of testing the fitness of persons to practise as dentists, who may be desirous of being so examined and to grant certificates of such fitness'. On the 1st December of that same year, the Odontological Society opened the Dental Hospital of London (at 32 Soho Square) and, on 1st October 1859, the London School of Dental Surgery. Together they formed the first dental training school in the United Kingdom.

The Act was updated with the 1921 Dentists Act, which made it obligatory that all those permitted to practise dentistry must have completed a specified course of training and passed the necessary examinations. Provision was made to allow those who had already practised dentistry for a specified period to continue so to do, exempt from these requirements, but anyone who did not fulfil these obligations was liable to be prosecuted. Many such cases did indeed come before the courts.

The result of the Act was to create two classes of dentists, the pre-1921 dentists, who had not studied for a qualification or passed the required examinations, and the post-1921 dental surgeons who had studied for the four-year course to obtain their qualifications. It was well into the 1950s before all the former had retired.

Since 1921 there have been other Acts which have affected the profession, such as those making provision for dental hygienists, dental auxiliaries, and other auxiliary helpers.

On 12th March 1874, the hospital and school moved to 40 Leicester Square (the site later occupied by the Leicester Square Cinema), a building that had, for a number of years, housed the Leicester Square soup kitchen! It was suitably altered and adapted. Particular attention was paid to the architectural treatment of the façade, with the intention that it would represent a 'noble and impressive elevation which, in so conspicuous position, could not fail to lead to more exalted estimation of the institution and profession it represents'. Over time, however, it became more and more obvious that a purpose built building was a desirable and so, after much deliberation and searching, a new site was found at 32 Leicester Square, the new establishment opening in 1901. This was where I trained.

This progression of events was not achieved without considerable disagreement amongst those promoting the cause of dentistry, not the least of which were the issues of raising funds for the building and the funding of patients' treatment. It was still largely an age when the extraction of teeth and the provision of dentures were the main treatments and both the design of the building and the dental syllabus reflected this.

Although the school was admitted to the University of London in 1911, and the degree of Bachelor of Dental Surgery of the university offered from 1920 onwards, it was not until 1934 that students for this degree were admitted to the school. The main reason for this was that it was still being maintained by many within the profession, that the Licentiate in Dental Surgery of the Royal College of Surgeons of England (LDS, RCS, Eng.) covered all the requirements for the practice of dentistry. They held the view that those wishing to gain further knowledge and advancement should obtain a medical qualification as well. This was encouraged by reducing the overall undergraduate period for those combining the two qualifications.

The dental course in 1938 was very different to that of today and still seemed to be based on the requirement of the 1921 Act. Apart from lectures and demonstrations in anatomy and physiology, lectures in metallurgy, dental mechanics, and dental anatomy, the first two years were spent in the dental laboratory learning how to construct metal and vulcanite dentures, i.e. learning the trade of a dental technician. It was not until all the exercises were completed that we were allowed to see a patient. We then had to construct at least 20 full sets of upper and lower dentures and a number of partial dentures - with some gold dentures if we were lucky - following the whole process from the first chair side impression, right through to the fitting of the final prosthesis.

Acrylic was unknown in those days and so the main components of any dentures were vulcanised rubber and porcelain teeth. In hindsight, and later knowing something about the financial relationship between hospital and school, it seems obvious that one of the reasons for this laboratory training was that the students thus contributed towards the small charge made to patients for their dentures - the maximum charge being £5 for full upper and lower dentures (many were unable to afford this and some paid less following the almoner's assessment). The examination taken at the end of these first two years had a practical element based on the exercises completed at the beginning of the course, plus the setting up and completion of dentures (not involving patients in this case). It also required written papers and oral examinations to be taken in the other subjects.

There was no CU at RDH but, as our anatomy and physiology courses were held at King's College, Strand, we were able to attend their CU meetings on the days that we had lectures there. Edwin Haigh, from CLS, was also a student there for the first part of his medical course. Another person I met there was Donald Wiseman, who eventually became a professor and wrote many Christian books. This CU was a section of the London Inter-Faculty Christian Union (LIFCU), one of the constituents of the Inter-Varsity Fellowship (IVF), renamed in the 1950s the University and Colleges Christian Fellowship (UCCF). Another attraction of studying at King's was the cheap lunch in the refectory - a two course luncheon with coffee was only 7d.

Even as I began my training as a dental surgeon, war clouds were gathering. With the knowledge of the devastation caused by air attacks in the Spanish Civil War, British civilians were being encouraged to train as air raid wardens, first aid workers, and the like, and to form the ARP organisations. After attending lectures at the local council offices, my mother and I were some of the first to obtain our warden certificates. We then helped to organise subsequent courses. In June 1939, everyone in the country was issued with a gas mask.

During that summer it became more and more apparent that we were on the brink of war. Whilst I was at the Bembridge Pioneer camp, Isle of Wight, the threat seemed so imminent that we discussed at our officer meetings whether we should strike camp early. In the end we decided against such action.

Whilst I was at camp my father and mother had to leave our house at Hinchley Wood and moved to a first floor flat in Leytonstone, East London, owned by Uncle Horace. It was rather small and dismal but we remained there until 1941 when my mother moved to Kirkby, near Liverpool, to join my father at the farmhouse provided for him by the MoS on his appointment as stores manager at their new royal ordnance factory.

On the last day of August I received a telegram from RDH saying, "If war declared hospital closed await instructions". So the uncertainty and anxieties of war were upon us.

Ready for Anything!

War was declared on 3rd September 1939. The first eight months were fairly uneventful, both from a national viewpoint and from our family perspective. Life did change in some respects, however, with the issuing of identity cards and ration books, for example, the fitting of special headlight deflectors to all motor vehicles, and the ruling that only one dim blue light was allowed in each train compartment, although later improved blackout which allowed more light to shine within the compartments was fitted to the carriages. No lights at all were allowed to show from houses, offices and shops. Travelling at night became difficult but everyone soon adapted to blackout conditions.

On the declaration of war the RDH was closed, as forewarned in the telegram, but only remained so for a few days. I spent this time driving my father around Surrey and nearby counties so that he could visit factories and similar establishments to sell air raid shelters - I think he worked on a commission basis.

My studies soon resumed and on my return I was advised that, as a special wartime concession, I could sit the dental mechanics practical examination (first professional examination) almost immediately - four months ahead of schedule. This gave little time for any instruction or revision in the various exercises vital to the examination, and unfortunately, I failed. The next examination was in January 1940, the date I had originally been scheduled to sit it. I took it again and this time passed. During these four months of further revision I sat next to Raymond Bird in the mechanics laboratory. This was the beginning of a lifelong friendship that has continued until his death in 2006.

I then commenced the 'phantom head' class where, for the next three months, we prepared cavities in extracted teeth which had been mounted in a simulated skull. Into the cavities we then inserted either amalgam or synthetic fillings. For these three months we were only able to use treadle drill machines, although the RDH was equipped, unlike most other dental schools, with electric drills. All students taking their finals in London had to take a treadle engine with them. I had to use one in my finals practical examination.

For the next 18 months we had to complete a stipulated number of fillings for patients including gold inlays and other types of restorations, undertake dresserships in the gas and surgical clinics and various other departments of the hospital, and attend certain courses of lectures as specified by the royal colleges.

There were a number of problems associated with wartime conditions, the major one being the shortage of patients. This was partly due to the population of London having dwindled considerably and partly because those sections of the public who regularly had treatment at the hospital were unable to be absent from their important war work during the daytime. There was also a lack of children, so many of them having been evacuated.

Every evening, and when we had a daytime air raid warning, we had to carry our dental cabinets, full of instruments, from the fifth floor to the basement, so that they would not be damaged if bombs fell on the building. During the London blitz, lecturers were quite often unable to honour their timetables because they had duties in other hospitals attending to air raid casualties.

When one had ARP warden duties, or had to spend the night in an air raid shelter, study at home became almost impossible. One tried to study on the daily journey to and from Leicester Square but that time was often spent catching up on missed sleep. Life was not easy.

Our first floor flat at 20 Queens Road, Leytonstone, left much to be desired. It was in a very run-down condition, had no hot running water and only a gas ring for cooking, although we did have an oil stove as well. It was also damp and cold. There was a bathroom but, with the lack of hot water, we had to walk up to my Uncle Horace's house at 24 Wallwood Road, for baths. The flat did later prove to have one advantage in that, when the gas mains were hit during the London blitz and gas supplies were cut-off, we could at least cook on our oil stove ring!

Before bomb damage made this impossible, I travelled into central London each day on the LNER suburban steam-hauled train to Liverpool Street and then the London underground to Leicester Square - the extension of the Central London underground line was not completed until after the war (the partly completed tunnels were used as air raid shelters).

My mother was appointed a full-time salaried ARP warden at Post 21, located in a glade on the edge of Wanstead Flats opposite St Andrews Church, the various ARP and first aid qualifications she had obtained before the outbreak of hostilities no doubt making her a good candidate for the job. Her salary was so small that it was not taxable and she had to work eight-hour shifts. I became a part-time, non-salaried ARP warden, attached to the same post. My duties were at night times and weekends. As I had also obtained my certificate 'A' during my time in the CLS OTC, I was automatically on the reserve of potential army officers and was called in for an interview at South Kensington. However, when it was realised that I was in a reserved occupation (providing I did not fail any professional examination more than once!), I was sent home again.

Around November or December of that year, my father successfully applied for an executive appointment with the MoS (royal ordnance) and was appointed for training to Chester-le-Street, near Durham. He came home at Christmas and on a few long weekends, but I am sure that the train journey was never very comfortable. The family had the usual Christmas celebrations at my Uncle's house in Wallwood Road, Leytonstone. Everyone was present, including my cousin Bill (who, being in the TA had been mobilised on the outbreak of war), but this was the last Christmas that we were all together - the end of an era.

* * * * *

London University was now scattered throughout the country, students in the various faculties joining with those of other universities in locations where it was considered that air raids were less likely. This meant that LIFCU gatherings in all but the medical and dental schools were likewise scattered, students being encouraged to support their adopted university CU. Two or three of us at RDH met in the museum of the hospital during the lunch hour, although on a somewhat irregular basis. Douglas Johnson, the then secretary of the IVF, sometimes joined us as a guest speaker. Soon even these meetings had to be curtailed with lunch breaks becoming shorter and shorter due to the hospital having to closing quite early during the winter months. This was necessary due to the impossibility of blacking out the vast conservatory type windows, particularly the overhead ones at the top of the building in the conservation department.

It seems that we made some impact on the school secretariat for, following the sudden death in1948 of Dean, Professor Harry Stobie, I was asked to organise the stewarding at his memorial service at St Martin's-in-the-Fields, Trafalgar Square, the hospital's parish church. By this time I was on the staff of the hospital myself.

It was also in these early days of the war that I became involved in various student activities within the hospital; this really stemmed from the time I was asked to organise a national savings group, part of the nationwide national savings campaign enabling members to purchase pre-dated national savings certificates. Shortly after this I was asked to be secretary of the Joint Planning Committee of Dental Students (JPCDS). We published two reports, the last in 1942, and these are available in the British Library and the library of the British Dental Association (BDA). Many of the recommendations can be seen in the development of post-war dental training and organisation. Was it a coincidence that, within a year of the last of these reports being published, the medical committee of the school set up a special subcommittee 'to consider the best scheme for the school and hospital in the post-war period'? The chairman of this committee was the Dean, Professor H. Stobie. The other members were Messrs. Ainsworth, Greenish, Bowdler-Henry, and Packham, all of whom were honorary dental surgeons and part-time teachers at the school.

The JPCDS was formed, by London dental students, because problems of wartime travelling made it impossible for students from the provinces to travel into London. Various questionnaires were sent to the student bodies in the provincial dental schools and at a provincial meeting, which was held in Manchester in early 1942, it was decided to form a British Dental Students Association (BDSA) of which I, as a founder member, was elected as vice-president a few months later. For a period after the cessation of hostilities the BDSA developed political overtones, an eventuality that was never envisaged by its founder members. These problems were eventually overcome and, until it was finally swallowed up by the BDA, the society was a vigorous, thriving organisation.

Camping was out of the question in wartime but in August 1940, a house party for former Pioneer campers and their friends was held at Gadebridge Park School, Hemel Hempstead, Hertfordshire. There were one or two daytime air raid alerts towards the end of this 'camp' and we used to watch aircraft taking off from nearby airfields, not at this time realising the devastation that was to come in the months to follow. I travelled back with David Tryon (the camp commandant), sharing the car with all the equipment. We drove to his offices in Wimbledon and I continued home by train to Leytonstone the following day. That night there was an air raid warning and we slept underneath the strong board room table at the headquarters of the South Africa General Mission (SAGM) all night. (The SAGM later became the African Evangelical Fellowship, the parent body of Pioneer camps.)

The Battle of Britain, fought in the skies over southern England for the next few weeks, brought only minor interruption to hospital duties with daytime air raid warnings. The London blitz opened up in all its fury on the first Saturday afternoon in September. My mother was on duty in a large communal air raid shelter on Wanstead Flats and I joined her there. No bombs were dropped near us, but at the London docks a few miles away, bombs fell on the *Tate & Lyle* sugar factory and various warehouses. When the all clear sounded we could see the fires burning fiercely in these areas, giving a clear indication of targets for the bombers returning at night. The sirens sounded again at dusk and bombing continued all night, the all clear not sounding until dawn.

During the following week there were many daylight raids as well as those at night. The daylight raids then stopped, but from then on until early in 1941 there were constant night raids, with just a short respite over Christmas. This made life very difficult and dental studies almost impossible as I had to combine nightly air raid warden patrols around Leytonstone with fire watchers duties at the RDH. I was lucky if I managed four hours sleep each night. Needless to say, the spirit of the East End Londoners was magnificent, as each night at dusk, they came up to our shelter on trolley buses or other transport. There would be a whole row of trolley buses parked along the Whipps Cross Road; drivers, conductors, and passengers would 'sleep' in the shelter and then go back to the East End of London again as soon as the all clear sounded next morning, many to find their homes destroyed during the night - we heard many sad stories.

The bringing of the buses out of central London was looked upon favourably by *London Transport,* for it meant that they were in a relatively safe area overnight and remained undamaged. They were thus able to stay in operation during a difficult period and, equally important, the *London Transport* staff were kept safe from injury.

Incidents during the blitz were numerous and it is not possible to recall them all. One I remember particularly well, which happened early on, was when an unexploded bomb fell on the path opposite our flat at 20 Queens Road. We were not allowed to return to the flat for several days and this resulted in mother and I living with the twins in Uncle Horace's house (24 Wallwood Road), Uncle and Auntie having evacuated to Aspley Guise as soon as the bombing started.

Our flat became uninhabitable so we stayed with the twins until mother was able to move to Kirkby, near Liverpool, to be with my father. I then went to live with John Ruff in Carshalton, Surrey. Our living with twins pleased Uncle and Auntie, and my father, as they knew that we would look after each other and report on all the happenings. When we were not on duty, we slept in the basement under the billiard table. I had a camp bed against a strengthened wall. It is amazing what you can become accustomed to and even Taffy, our dog, took it all in his stride.

Uncle Horace owned a lot of property in and around Leytonstone, some of which was rented to quite elderly tenants. Quite often windows were blown out during raids and other damage sustained. My cousin Bill was still in camp with his unit in Essex but was able to come home some weekends. Between us we did what temporary repairs we could to the houses.

Early in the blitz, the railway line into Liverpool Street was damaged and very soon travel by train into London became impossible. To cope with the problem of getting people to work, express services were introduced on several bus routes around London during morning and evening rush hours - you could only board these buses at certain set points in the suburbs and only alight at the central London terminus, and vice versa in the evenings. Tickets for this service were very cheap; much cheaper than using a rail season ticket. Such a route, the one we used, was number 38. We boarded the bus at Bakers Arms, about 15 minutes walk from Wallwood Road, and alighted close to the British Museum, from where one could walk to the RDH at Leicester Square.

When several London bus garages, and the buses in them, were destroyed in the blitz, buses from the provinces were drafted into London. They retained their various liveries, bringing back memories of the 'pirate' buses much favoured during the years we lived in East Sheen.

Fire watching at the hospital was quite an experience. Every building in London had to have its fire watchers, the duties usually performed, after some basic training, by the staff of offices, departmental stores, etc. The role of a fire watcher was to extinguish the small incendiary bombs dropped by enemy aircraft before the fire had a chance to take hold and potentially engulf the building. It was a vitally important job. At the RDH, students, nurses, and clerical staff shared these duties. We usually worked in pairs - I teamed up with Raymond Bird - and there was a room set aside in the basement for those on duty. It contained bunk beds and facilities for cooking light meals and making copious cups of tea.

During raids, we patrolled the building, paying particular attention to the flat roof, to ensure that if any incendiary bombs were dropped, we could extinguish them using the stirrup pump before they did any damage. You certainly had a very good view of the whole of south London from the roof of our building. Fortunately no bombs were dropped on the Royal and the only damage was to windows from blast from bombs dropped on other property in the vicinity.

A landmine, a huge container of high explosive dropped by parachute that detonated on impact, fell on the billiard saloon in Panton Street, off Leicester Square. It happened on the 16th October. Every pane of glass in our building was broken and the lift put out of action. Fortunately Raymond and I were not on duty that night but those who were on duty were blown out of their beds and badly shaken.

With the top floor of the building having a glass roof, there was a considerable quantity of glass to be cleared; it was a case of all hands to the pump for staff and students, the glass being swept into dustbins and then tipped out of the windows into the street below. It was then carted away by the City of Westminster staff; no complaints by anyone in those days as all worked to the common good of keeping London moving.

I was doing my general anaesthetics dressership that month and I remember that we had emergency services in operation the following day. By the beginning of the following week, all departments were working normally, the emergency repairs to windows and fabric having been completed by then.

It was during these months that the devotion to duty of the resident head porter, Jack Knight (who had suffered from shell-shock in the First World War), and his wife, was greatly appreciated, especially for their kindness to those on night duty during the blitz. He was an elder of the small non-conformist chapel in the road behind the hospital, Orange Street Congregational Chapel, and they both had a sound Christian faith.

By February 1941, my father was established in his appointment at the newly completed Royal Ordnance Factory at Kirkby on the outskirts of Liverpool. The requisitioned farmhouse he was allocated, Moses Farm, was on the perimeter road around the site, about 2 miles from the main entrance. He travelled backwards and forwards to work by bicycle, which was also his main means of transport in and around the factory, a largely hutted establishment.

Once my father had settled in, my mother moved from Leytonstone to join him. I saw her off from Euston station, complete with bicycle and dog, and my father met her at Lime Street, Liverpool and they proceeded by MoS transport to Moses Farm, Kirkby, their new home. The household contents followed by removal van later. At this time there was no direct local public transport from the centre of Liverpool to the factory - one had to proceed by tram and change to a special bus for the last part of the journey. Later the tramslines were extended to the factory gates and one then had to cycle to Moses Farm.

I now took up residence with fellow Pioneer camper and dental student, John Ruff (who was training at the National Dental Hospital, Great Portland Street), and his mother, they having kindly invited me to live with them at their home in Carshalton, Surrey. John's father had recently died and his elder brother was a prisoner of war in Italy.

The weekend before Easter, I took our car, which had been garaged at Wallwood Road, to *Gates Motors* at Woodford for servicing and then on Maunday Thursday, drove it all the way to Kirkby. This was no mean feat as there were no road signs, all of them having been removed when threat of invasion loomed following the occupation of mainland Europe by the German armies. Putting my good map reading skills to work (learnt when I was in the OTC), I had an uneventful journey, but it was 'seat of the pants' driving, reliant on us knowing that Liverpool was north-north-west of London! It was with much relief to everyone, particularly my mother's, that I arrived safely.

The car would prove to be most useful to both my mother and my father, living right out in the heart of the country as they did; Kirkby was just a small village in those days, not the massive new town development it is today. Their petrol ration was meagre but it did enabled them to get to Kirkby Station, from where there were several trains each day to Liverpool Exchange or Wigan (where my mother's friend from East Sheen had been evacuated). The car also got them to church at Knowsly (Lord Derby's estate) on Sundays.

About five miles distant from Kirkby was the market town of Ormskirk. A similar distance away was St Helens, where my parents soon made friends with one of my father's business acquaintances. Southport (where we could obtain special items with my forces ration card), could be easily reached by the frequent electric train service from Liverpool Exchange, the journey taking less than an hour. It was also possible to visit Chester for the day by train from other Liverpool stations.

In the Summer of 1941, a Pioneer house party was held at Stamford School, Rutland. The actual cooking was undertaken by the school staff, under the supervision of the headmaster's wife, but I had the task of dealing with all the ration books and obtaining the appropriate supplies from the local shops. This proved to be quite a nightmare but everyone, including the headmaster's wife, seemed to be quite happy and thought that I had worked miracles!

Whilst shopping in the town one day, whom should we meet but Geoff Baker, one of the officers from the North Wales VPS camps of the mid-30s. He was an Ealing Crusader leader and I had seen him on several occasions at Crusader gatherings; he was now an army officer stationed locally.

Around this time, the Church Missionary Society (CMS) were making a recruitment film. Their plans to film some of the sequences in one of the London medical schools had to be abandoned because so many of the students had been evacuated elsewhere. It was at this point that I was approached by Mr Lomax, their visual aids secretary, he being aware of my interest in the society, mainly through my cousin Dick (Wootton) I believe. The outcome was an arrangement that they would film a mock lecture in the RDH lecture theatre and that one of the students would attend at CMS headquarters near Ludgate Circus to pose as a candidate for the overseas mission field for the next sequence of the film. This was duly accomplished and so the Royal appeared on celluloid for many years thereafter.

My new home at 15 Salisbury Road, Carshalton, was equidistant from Carshalton and Carshalton Beeches stations. A season ticket enabled you to travel from either of these stations to any *London Southern Railway* terminus, with trains terminating at either London Bridge (with direct access to Charing Cross, a few minutes' walk to the dental hospital) or Victoria. It could not have been a more convenient venue.

I continued as an ARP warden in Carshalton Beeches. Duties were less arduous and less frequent now that the regular nightly alerts had ceased. Sundays proved to be a very busy day - John and I usually attended morning service at Sutton Baptist Church, then cycled up to Banstead (a very uphill journey) in the afternoon where we were both assistant leaders of the Banstead Crusader class (leader, Terence Fuller). If there was no Crusader class committee meeting or other Crusader function following the afternoon class, we then attended the evening service at Morden Parish Church (vicar, Rev Jack Ainley). It was not practicable to arrange week-night meetings of leaders due to wartime restrictions, wartime duties, and my undergraduate studies.

Eventually I took over charge of the junior section of the Banstead Class. The Crusader classes in the area held a house party during the school summer holidays at Abbey School (a boarding school just south of East Grinstead). We cycled there on the middle Saturday to visit our own members attending this summer event.

My lasting memory of the evening service Morden Parish Church is that, whilst still kneeling after the blessing at the end of the service we quietly sang the hymn:

> *May the mind of Christ our Saviour,*
> *And the Father's boundless love,*
> *With the Holy Spirit's favour,*
> *Rest upon us from above.*
> *Thus may we abide in union*
> *With each other and the Lord.*
> *And possess, in sweet communion,*
> *Joys which earth cannot afford.*

And then we went out into the blackout and all the dangers of a wartime night.

* * * * *

There was a Sutton Crusader Fellowship that met once a month on a Saturday evening in the Sutton Crusader Hall, and occasionally (more regularly once I had qualified and evening revision was no longer a necessity), I was able to attend the mid-week meeting at Morden Parish Church. When I was called up for the navy I continued to have contact with the class, visiting them on Sundays when I had a short weekend leave, and editing the Banstead Crusader class forces newsletter until I left these shores to join the British Pacific Fleet.

Travel between Liverpool Lime Street and Euston during these years left much to be desired and so it was really only worthwhile if one could stay for a week or more at Kirkby. We always obtained a seat on the journey north but rarely on the return journey when we often had to travel in the guard's van. On one occasion, the train was so crowded that we were packed in the guard's van like sardines all the way from Liverpool to London, a journey which, due to the many hold-ups *en route*, could take as long as six hours.

I qualified as a dental surgeon in June 1942. I should have taken up a house surgeon appointment immediately but unfortunately, I contracted chickenpox during the clinical part of finals through contact with a child who had the virus; I suffered very little from this illness but my father developed shingles and was on the sick list for several weeks. It was July before I was able to take up my new position.

One of the clinical examiners at my finals was 'Freddie' Doubleday of Guy's. Later, when I was organising the clinical patients at a subsequent finals examination (part of my role as house surgeon) I was amazed when he discussed with me the complete dental history of the patient I had examined in my own finals exam. On his retirement several years later, Mr Doubleday was ordained and appointed curate at Dorking Parish Church as a non-stipendiary minister.

It was shortly before my finals that I learnt (through the grapevine developed with the secretariat of the BDA from JPCDS contacts) there were now vacancies in the dental branch of the Royal Navy and I managed, after a few telephone calls, to transfer my preference for call-up to the senior service (I was originally registered for the RAF dental branch). I had an interview with the Director General (Dental), Rear Admiral Holgate and, following the usual medical, was accepted for the navy.

In the December of that year I was approached by the hospital representative of the *Amalgamated Dental Company*, the company which supplied the equipment for the dental surgery at the Royal Ordinance Factory. Having heard of me through my father, the representative was enquiring as to whether I could undertake a short locum for a Preston dental surgeon, Mr P.A. Gardner, who had to be hospitalised for a few weeks; his surgery was at his residence in Garstang Road. The Director General (Dental) of the navy agreed to this and so my call-up was delayed until February 1943.

So for the next few weeks, I worked midday Monday to midday Saturday each week in Preston, living in the Gardner's flat above the practice, then returned home by train to Kirkby, via Wigan, on Saturday afternoon, returning back to Preston on the first train on Monday morning - local train services and connections were more reliable in wartime than they are today! The experience was valuable and opened my eyes to the advantages and disadvantages of private dental practice and the problems of dealing with patients in such an environment; it also introduced me to the intricacies of the 'dental letter' system, whereby members of Provident Societies could claim part of the cost of their dental treatment from their respective society. This system continued until the introduction of the National Health Service (NHS) in 1948. Mr Gardner was eventually able to resume seeing his patients and so I returned to Kirkby to await instructions to join the Royal Navy.

Royal Navy

I joined the Royal Navy at RNB Devonport (*HMS Drake*) on 26th February1943, having travelled to Plymouth by the direct train service from Liverpool, via Shrewsbury and Hereford. The uniform I had ordered from *Messrs Gieves* in Liverpool followed me a few days later. My commission was temporary Surgeon Lieutenant (D), but after successfully completing a six month probationary period, a permanent commission was confirmed.

The first fortnight was one of basic training; how to march, how to salute, sword drill, etc. We also had talks on various naval customs and privileges, naval etiquette, naval accounting, and the like, followed by a gas course the following week. I then spent a week in the dental department learning about the various records that had to be completed, inspecting drafts when joining and leaving ship, and similar procedures. After spending some days in the dental department I went on a long weekend leave - Friday lunchtime to Monday evening (extra time being allowed for travelling for those living a long way from their ship).

Travel was now much more pleasant as, being a naval officer, I had to travel first class; we also qualified for special HM Forces fare concessions. When I returned on the Monday evening I was informed that I was 'on loan' to *HMS Raleigh*, a shore based establishment just across the Tamar at Torpoint, and I proceeded there the following day. This was my first insight to providing routine dental treatment for royal naval personnel. Wren mess stewards trained here and provided an excellent service in the mess. They also gave special attention to the officer's uniforms, sponging and pressing them each day.

On the Thursday, I received a signal instructing myself and my fellow dental officer, John Drury, to join *HMS Collingwood* at

Fareham, Hampshire. John was still accommodated at RNB and so I headed back to Plymouth and the following day we travelled by train to Fareham, the nearest station to Collingwood. There was a daily train service between Plymouth and Portsmouth.

HMS Collingwood was one of the navy's main initial training establishments, with an entry of 2,000 new recruits every fortnight. The initial training course lasted for eight weeks. There were 13 dental surgeries, plus one for the Surgeon Commander (D), but as there were more than 13 dental officers it was necessary to have a 'double banking' system whereby two dental officers worked in the same surgery, one team working from 0800-1500 Monday to Friday, the other team from 1500-1930 Monday to Friday and all day on Saturday. The system suited those who were married and lived ashore (i.e. not within the establishment) but was not so popular with others.

Every new recruit had to have a dental inspection and be rendered 'dentally fit' before the end of the eight weeks, so we were kept very busy providing routine dental treatment. I would estimate that, on average, every recruit needed five fillings and one extraction, the mouths of some being so bad that they needed a clearance at the age of 18 - a sad reflection of the dental health of the nation. Dentures were fitted at the recruit's next establishment but it was unlikely that those with full upper and lower dentures would ever serve at sea.

HMS Collingwood was a hutment establishment and extended over a very wide area. Nearly every officer, and other ranks on the permanent staff, had a bicycle for riding around the base and for visits within the Portsmouth command, and occasionally further afield. We were fortunate in having a large Royal Marine band for playing at Divisions (a formal parade service held Monday to Friday mornings for the whole ship's company). Their orchestra also provided music for the Sunday morning service which took place in the very large cinema (seating capacity of some 2000), and for stage productions and other more formal occasions such as ward room functions.

I spent almost two years on *HMS Collingwood* and it proved to be a very good introduction to the Royal Navy, both from the dental aspect and service in general. John Drury and I shared a cabin. He had trained at Guy's, was a very keen sportsman and had also served on the JPCDS with me.

When I entered the wardroom on the first evening, I noted that there was a letter pigeon-hole for Alan Brown and wondered if this was the same Alan Brown I knew as the leader of the Wallington Crusader Class (whom I met at the Sutton Crusader Fellowship) and a solicitor in the *Goodman, Goodman, Goodman, and Brown* partnership. It was! Although he was rarely in the mess himself, as he lived ashore with his wife and family, he introduced me to Sub-Lieutenant T.W.O. (Will) Matheson, an Irishman whose father was the Solicitor General for Eire, and whose company and Christian friendship I enjoyed throughout my time in Fareham. We became lifelong friends - I attended his wedding and two years later he, his wife, and young child, attended ours.

Will was a hockey international, which meant he was often away on Saturdays during the winter months either playing for his country's team, for the Royal Navy or for the Portsmouth Command. He was a good shove-halfpenny and billiard player! Like myself, Will was also a Crusader, and between us we unofficially 'welcomed' Crusaders undertaking their initial training on *Collingwood*. Once we became known to them, Crusader HQ alerted us to the names of Crusaders about to join *Collingwood*; if they were not in Will's Division, where it was his duty to interview all recruits, then we invited them to come to my dental surgery (not for dental treatment!) on an evening when they were off-duty. Here we were able to talk to them and put them at their ease - I first met one of my future brothers-in-law in this way!

We had good relationships with the navy chaplains, with only one exception, and on several occasions I was asked to represent the ship's company at a confirmation service for one or more of the trainees, which took place in the chapel at the nearby Bishop's Palace - those who had not been confirmed in their home church often felt the need to be confirmed (a spiritual safety net in some way I suppose) before facing the fear of death in a wartime situation. The padre conducted regular preparation classes which had to be attended before the candidate could be confirmed. One of the candidates, towards the end of my duties on *Collingwood*, was a fellow dental officer, Vic Simons, and I kept in touch with him over many years, later becoming godfather to his eldest son.

After I had been at *Collingwood* for about nine months, I was asked to serve on the Wardroom committee, in charge of newspapers and tobacco. This gave me another insight into naval customs; contacts with NAAFI stores made me aware of the dependence of the forces on their support.

It was shortly after this time that I was invited to be the naval representative on the Council of the Public Dental Services Association; their Lordships graciously agreeing to this. I also instituted courses of lectures on oral hygiene for each recruit intake, using film strips and models that were available from The Dental Board of the United Kingdom. There were no Dental Hygienists in the navy in these days. I wrote my first casual communication (on the subject of a large dental cyst of the right maxilla) during these years and this was published in the *Dental Record* (D. Gaz. 11.26. Sept 1944). Anyone reading this now will appreciate what advances have been made in dental science over the past 60 years.

A few months after I arrived in Fareham, I was asked if it would be possible for Will, myself, and others, to provide cover for the Sunday afternoon Covenanter class that was attached to Stubbington Parish Church, as the current leader, a civilian scientist with duties at the Fleet Air Arm at Lee-on-Solent, was moving to another part of the country. Although it was not possible to be present every week, we did our best; not an ideal situation but better than closing the class.

Will was an acknowledged lay preacher and visited non-conformist churches and gospel halls once a month on average. I often accompanied him and led the service, with Will giving the Address. On at least two occasions we cycled to the Crusader class at Petersfield as the leader, Robert Ewan, a great friend of Will's family, had invited him to speak at a birthday service or similar parent attended gathering.

Some Sunday evenings we worshipped at a small gospel hall at Peel Common, a few minutes cycle-ride from *Collingwood*, usually staying on for a hymn singing session after the service. At 2045 sharp they always sang 'Eternal Father strong to save' and prayed for all those who had trained at *Collingwood* and were serving in HM ships in the many theatres of war. Will and I occasionally visited Mr Munday, the missioner, at his home on a weekday evening. We played snooker with him on his full-size table and Monopoly with the rest of the family afterwards.

Although there had been some enemy air action before my arrival, all was quiet during most of my appointment. At one stage, there were early morning alerts for doodlebugs (V1 rockets) passing close by and presumably aimed at Southampton docks. On another occasion, a bomb jettisoned by an enemy aircraft to lighten its load in order to gain height after a raid elsewhere, fell on one of the Nissen huts causing several fatalities and other casualties.

We enjoyed much Christian fellowship in the Portsmouth area. The Army Scripture Reader at Gosport, Mr Hitchcock, held a fellowship evening in his house every Monday and Will Matheson and I would cycle over there when we were free. Will also introduced me to another Gosport family, Mrs Rankin and her children Moyra and Alwyn, who kept an 'open house' for the many service personnel serving in the area. Mr Rankin had also been an Army Scripture Reader, but had died shortly before I arrived in Fareham. We enjoyed their company, although our commitments were such that we usually only managed to visit on the occasional Saturday or Sunday afternoon.

One of the visitors to this home was John Prince, who had recently joined the navy and, after completing his training in Canada was commissioned in the Fleet Air Arm. After the war he married Moyra; it was a great wedding at Richmond, Surrey, a reunion of many friends of wartime years, with a guard of honour in true naval tradition provided by former officer colleagues. John and Moyra emigrated to Australia after he had completed a science degree at Downing College, Cambridge, and we have continued regular correspondence to this day. In 1948, some of us met together for a weekend at the newly formed Hildenborough Conference Centre in Kent when a Fellowship, the Rankinites, was formed.

It is of interest to note that even in wartime, the question of future peacetime activities was often discussed, especially how those trained as pilots and observers could use this knowledge in full-time Christian service. Those who trained in the Royal Air Force had similar visions and it was from these prayerful ideas that the Missionary Aviation Fellowship (now the Mission Aviation Fellowship) was formed. Its original concept was to transport missionaries and their supplies, and provide an emergency medical service, to remote locations on the continent of Africa which, by road or on foot, would have taken days if not weeks to reach. The mission has now developed, with many more aircraft available and it has extended its service to many parts of the world, working in cooperation with many mission organisations.

The Portsmouth and district branch of the Officer's Christian Union (OCU) also held monthly meetings in the Hitchcock's home; Captain Godfrey Buxton RA, the OCU general secretary, sometimes attended. One OCU member who attended a meeting shortly before D-Day, was Rev Maurice Wood, a naval chaplain, who was eventually to become principal of Oak Hill Theological Training College, North London, before being appointed Bishop of Norwich. Captain Buxton visited *Collingwood* once to address an assembly of officers and to distribute free copies of the *New Testament* to any who requested one.

Whilst at Collingwood, I was fortunately near enough to London to enable me to travel there for short weekend leaves (midday Saturday to Sunday evening) when I often stayed with Terence and Joan Fuller. This was very useful as it enabled me to edit the Banstead Crusaders Forces Newsletter; how much we appreciated the duplicating skills of Mrs B. Crossley of Parkstone, Dorset. I also spent some weekends at Bush Hill Park with Uncle Charlie and Auntie Edie, and others at Bexleyheath with Granny Mohr and Auntie Cissie.

* * * * *

The writing of this history has made me very aware of part of a verse in the Old Testament - 'I being in the way, the Lord led me' (Gen. 24 v27). In this chapter of the Bible, Abraham has sent his eldest servant into his own country to find a wife for Abraham's son Isaac. The servant asks God to guide him and make it plain to him when he had found the right girl, and this he does at the well in Nahor. How often seemingly chance circumstances bring us to a place where we are able to help others and have fellowship with them. Are they really chance or is God at work? I mention this at this point because of a situation that arose towards the end of our time in the Portsmouth area. Mr and Mrs Hitchcock were very concerned because their son David, who was only about a year old, had been diagnosed with a tumour behind his eye, the removal of which would almost certainly result in the loss of the eye. They asked us if we knew of a Christian consultant who could help them. It so happened that we knew a member of the Sutton Crusader Fellowship who was on the staff of one of the London teaching hospitals and we were able to put Mr Hitchcock in touch with him. He was able to treat David and reassure his parents.

D-Day meant increased activity for all the services in and around Portsmouth. Although our regular ship's company were not directly involved, some of our number, including Will Matheson, were loaned to Allied Command Headquarters, located in one of the forts in the hills behind Portsmouth, for several weeks before the actual landings in Normandy; this was mainly on a day to day basis for training, and then permanently just before the actual landings. They were engaged in plotting movements of ships and coordinating with all the forces involved in the landings. Our establishment became very overcrowded with officers for a short period before the big day. The officers included a number of old citizens and past schoolmates who were actually taking part in the landings, although mainly as beach party personnel.

For many weeks before the landings, troops were assembling in the area. When the wind was blowing in the right direction, lorries, upon which were mounted smoke producing vats, parked on the road outside our main gates and belched forth clouds of dark oily smoke with the help of rather noisy fans. This spread across the whole area, concealing troop movements and the crafts moored in the Solent and all around the dockyard. All leave was cancelled and everyone, naval personnel and civilians alike, had to obtain special passes if they needed to travel anywhere near the coast - I had to have one to travel to the Stubbington Covenantor class. All outgoing mail was heavily censored and telephone calls were not permitted.

We all knew when the first troops had landed, such was special naval intelligence, and on many occasions after that we stood and watched fleets of gliders passing overhead. These we knew to be carrying troops and equipment to support the ground forces.

Early in 1945, I was appointed to *HMHS Gerusalemme*, a naval hospital ship, as senior dental officer; I was actually the only dental officer on board! At the same time, one of my fellow dental officers, Vic Simons, whom I knew very well, received instructions to join *HMHS Vasna*. He had been 'secretly' engaged to a Chief Wren Petty Officer, our senior wardroom steward, for many months, and on receiving this appointment they got married. At the end of the war, when Vic's troopship was due to dock at Liverpool, his wife Marjorie stayed with my parents at Kirkby so that she could be at the dockside to greet him. Vic remained another lifelong friend. He made a cine-film at our wedding and I was godfather to his eldest son.

Vic and I left Fareham on embarkation leave at the same time, having been told to wait for notification of where we would be heading next. I received various instructions from the Ministry of War transport department advising me to contact them in a month if I had not received detailed instructions. Meanwhile, I was to have certain inoculations and obtain tropical rig.

Before I left *Collingwood* I had ascertained from the Radar School (who had records of all ship movements), that *Gerusalemme* was undergoing a refit in Cape Town and so I thought that this would be my destination. At the beginning of April, I received instructions to proceed to Gourock, Scotland, to join HMT J7. My father secured me a first class sleeper on the Liverpool to Glasgow train for the night before I was due to join the ship, and I then travelled on the local train to Gourock where I received my boarding pass for cabin LP7 and third sitting in the officers' mess for meals - there were about five sittings for every meal! I was transported by tender to a very large liner lying at anchor on the Clyde. She was the *SS Nieuw Amsterdam* of the *Holland American Line* and was captained by Captain Commander Barendse.

On boarding the ship, I discovered that I was bound for Australia. It later transpired that because the Ministry of War transport department had forgotten me, the *Gerusalemme* had left South Africa without me, hence the need for me to sail to Australia to join her. I was on board the *Nieuw Amsterdam* for five days before we set sail; security was such that a ship was 'sealed' for two days or longer before the voyage began, with no contact with the shore.

Troopships played an important role in both world wars, conveying large numbers of forces personnel to areas where fighting forces were needed. The *Nieuw Amsterdam* was an example of such a ship, she being the second in the *Holland-American Line* fleet to bear this famous name, the previous vessel having been launched in 1906 and laid up in 1930. Our vessel was built at Rotterdam and launched in 1937, Queen Wilhelmina performing the naming ceremony. She came into service on the North Atlantic route in May the following year.

When, in May 1940, Holland was forces to capitulate to Nazi Germany, *Nieuw Amsterdam* was on a short cruise in the Caribbean. On returning to New York, she was handed over to the British Ministry of Transport. All her luxurious fittings were stripped out and suitable equipment installed to prepare her for wartime use and with accommodation for many thousands of service personnel as possible. An example of this was that my cabin, which was originally a first class cabin with en-suite facilities, was now equipped with 18 bunks, arranged in tiers. The bathroom facilities remained the same!

Her crew stayed with her and served on her throughout the war, being unable to return to their homes which were occupied by the enemy. When peace was declared she conveyed many thousands of troops and civilians back to their homelands. By this time, she had travelled 530,652 miles as a troopship. Finally, she was able to return home herself, to be given a complete overhaul and replacement and update of her original fittings, once again becoming the pride of the *Holland-American Line*. She then continued to serve on the North Atlantic voyages until progress in air travel overtook the regular routes of sea travel and she became a cruise ship. Age eventually took their toll and *Nieuw Amsterdam* was sent to the scrap yard in 1974.

On the evening of 22nd April, our wait in port finally came to an end and the *Nieuw Amsterdam* weighed anchor and sailed down the Clyde out into open sea. For the first 24 hours we had an escort and adopted a zigzag course, resuming plain sailing until within a few hours of passing Gibraltar. We had a very pleasant and uneventful journey, rather cool for the first few days but warming sufficiently for us to change into tropical rig the day after entering the Mediterranean.

There were many naval personnel on board, all of us on our way to join the British Pacific Fleet, and also a number of Royal Australian Air Force personnel returning home after duties in Europe. This made for a very crowded ship. The food was generally very good, with three meals a day: breakfast - the usual; lunch - cold meat plus cake, cheese and coffee; supper - soup, a roast main course, and a sweet. Our afternoons were spent up on deck, during most of the voyage, but in the evenings the outer deck was out of bounds due to blackout regulations. Our evenings were thus spent in the saloon, which became very crowded. The other main problem on board was with water, both for drinking and washing, and it was only available for four hours each day. Sea water was available for baths in the early evening.

The dental department on board, which was situated in the beauty parlour, had the great advantage of being air-conditioned. It was equipped with an American field dental kit which, although quite good, contained few instruments of English pattern. I operated in the clinic in the mornings and Surg/Lt Watt RNVR, of MONAB 6, covered the afternoon. During the course of the voyage we treated some 250 cases, mainly emergencies.

The ship also had a good library and canteen. The latter sold many goods unobtainable in the UK, but they were mostly American and very expensive.

On Sunday mornings there were two church services, one at 1030 and the other at 1115, with community hymn singing on the open deck in the early evening before dark; all were well attended. For the first time I appreciated the significance of the hymn 'The day Thou gavest Lord is ended'. We were sailing east and I became very aware that it is always daytime in some part of the world and that the voice of prayer is never silent.

Our only port of call *en route* was at Suez, where we took on oil and water. On passing through the Red Sea the bareness of the land through which the 'Children of Israel' travelled was very apparent. At 1500 hours on May 16th, we docked at Fremantle, Western Australia. No shore leave was allowed but the following day a route march to the local stadium was arranged and we were greeted by the civic authorities with apples, biscuits, cake, milk and orangeade. A good time was had by all! We set sail again at 1500 the following day and at 1130 on 23rd May, docked at jetties six and seven at Woolloomooloo, Sydney. We should have arrived sooner but thick fog kept us outside the harbour boom for three or four hours.

The medical personnel on board the ship disembarked at 0945 the following day and travelled by bus to the Royal Naval Hospital at Herne Bay. Luggage followed later the same day but one case of mine, which was eventually found in a locked hut at the naval base, took three days to locate.

My accommodation at Herne Bay Hospital, a war-time hutted hospital spread over a large area on the outskirts of Sydney, was cabin 11 in hut 242. It contained only a bed and temporary wardrobe at first, although a table did arrive a few days later. Washing conditions left much to be desired; no washbasins and only a communal trough. Messing was good but very expensive. The dental surgery was very large but had only one dental chair. The dental officer there was assisted by two Red Cross nurses (VADs). I worked alternate watches with him.

The electrified railway system had been extended to within a short distance of the hospital gates and this provided a frequent fast service to the centre of Sydney, running over the underground system to the harbour terminus. I was only able to visit Sydney in the evenings and so was not able to see much of the city. I contacted the CSSM and a Miss Nicholson introduced me to *Everyman's* in George Street, a sort of YMCA for the forces, led by Gordon Issigard. I spoke at this club on Sunday evening, May 27th, and Sub/Lt/ Kennedy, who had travelled on the same troopship as myself and whom I had met unexpectedly on the previous evening, accepted a decision card from Mr Issigard.

* * * * *

We now learnt that *HMHS Gerusalemme* had docked in Melbourne and we made plans to join her there. We set off on June 1st, travelling on the 2045 train from Sydney Central Station. It was an overnight sleeper and I shared a two-berth compartment with another medical officer who was joining the ship. Due to an accident on the line the previous evening, the train did not actually depart until 0045. Because of the delay, a breakfast stop was made at Junce Junction. We all alighted from the train - passengers and railway staff (including the engine driver and fireman) - and all had a very substantial breakfast in the station buffet at the expense of the railway company. We then proceeded to Albury where we had to change trains because the rail gauge differed between the states of New South Wales and Victoria. We joined a new, very comfortable diesel streamlined train, *Spirit of Progress*, and, because the changeover was normally early morning, were served with a second breakfast instead of lunch! We arrived at Melbourne Spencer Street at 1600 hours.

The final leg of the journey, from the station to Port Melbourne where *Gerusalemme* was alongside, was by official transport. We arrived there at about 1800 hours. The duty medical officer for the day was Surg/Lt 'Charlie' Drew, the brother of one of my fellow students at RDH. I was directed to cabin 7 and, after dinner, was finally able to unpack and settle into my quarters. The following day, I received all the mail that had been piling up for me since I had left the UK (all the mail for the British Pacific Fleet came by air).

My first duty was to inspect the dental surgery which had been maintained by Sick Berth Petty Officer (D) Oakley since the ship left Cape Town. I also completed other routine duties required of any officer taking up a new appointment. I was informed that it had already been agreed that I should take on the role of ship's Film Officer, although at this point there was no projector, no films, or associated equipment on board!

I learnt that *Gerusalemme* was originally Benito Mussolini's Royal Yacht which the Italian navy had scuttled in the harbour at Lorenco Marques in rather shallow water. It had been floated by the South African navy and fitted-out as a hospital ship in Durban. Many defects had revealed themselves on the voyage from Africa to Australia and it had been necessary for the ship to dock in Albany, Western Australia, for various repairs but they were unable to attend to the inadequate refrigeration plant and so the ship proceeded to Melbourne for this work. It was estimated that it would take a fortnight, but it was five weeks before the required standard was achieved to enable us to serve in the tropics.

As with all hospital ships, navigation, engineering and catering staff, both officers and crew, were provided by the Merchant Navy and on our ship, they were employees of the *Union Castle Line*. Except for the Padre, a Supply Officer and his staff of two (who dealt with all naval finances and regulations), and a Yeoman of Signals and his assistants, all the other naval staff were medical, with eight specialist staff; myself, a Ward Master, Matron, six Nursing Sisters, and almost 100 Sick Berth Attendants (SBAs). As well as the dental surgery there was an X-Ray department, two operating theatres, a pathological laboratory, and accommodation for up to 450 patients in swinging beds or hammocks. All the senior officers were regular Royal Navy but about half of us were wartime Royal Navy Volunteer Reserves (RNVRs).

I was about to embark on a very interesting phase of my naval career...

The Forgotten Fleet

HMHS Gerusalemme was the hospital ship for the British Pacific Fleet, a part of the so-called 'Fleet Train'. This was a fleet of which little had been heard in the UK, including in naval circles. Yet on VJ Day in 1945, the combined British Pacific and East Indies Fleets had more than 600 ships and landing craft and nearly a quarter of a million personnel - British, Australians, New Zealanders, Canadians, Indians, and South Africans; the greatest commonwealth fleet in history. It had won the admiration and respect of our American allies and yet the fleet in the Far East was rarely, if ever, mentioned in the UK. Indeed, I would suggest that after VE-Day, the majority of the population in UK considered that all hostilities had ceased and gave no thought to the continued fighting in the Far East.

A Reviewer, John Winton, wrote in his book *The Forgotten Fleet*,

> When Admiral Sir Bruce Fraser hoisted his flag as Commander-in-Chief of the British Pacific Fleet (BPF) in November 1944, the United States navy had already won the important battles of the Philippine Sea and Leyte Gulf and was waging sea warfare across vast distances on a scale which the Royal Navy could not hope to equal. In the Pacific in 1945 the Royal Navy had therefore to learn, for the first time in its history, how to be a poor relation.
>
> The arrival of the British fleet in the Pacific was preceded by a long period of political controversy and American suspicion. The fleet faced enormous difficulties, of distance, of supply, and manpower. The Fleet Train, whose magnificent performance kept the fleet at sea, was a motley collection of tankers, store

and repair ships, which in general were too small, too slow, and too few. Despite generous American assistance, there were many shortages and deficiencies. Lack of fuel cruelly denied most of the BPF its proper right to be present at the final surrender of Japan in Tokyo Bay.

Yet the BPF, led at sea by Vice-Admiral Sir Bernard Rowlings, overcame every difficulty and, together with the East Indies Fleet under Admiral Sir Arthur John Power, went on to write new and stirring pages of naval history - in the air strikes on the Palembang oil refineries, in combined operations with the 14th Army in the Arakan, in their gallant behaviour under the terrifying attacks of kamikaze suicide bombers off the Sakishima Gunto, the capture of Rangoon and the sinking of *Haguro*, the daring penetrations of Singapore, Saigon and Hong Kong harbours by midget submarines, the attack on the Japanese home islands with Halsey's Third Fleet, and, finally, the landings in Malaya and the reoccupation of Singapore. After the surrender, the fleet was the only large mobile force immediately available for the repatriation of Commonwealth prisoners of war and internees, and the rehabilitation of former British territory in the Far East.

Not long after I joined the ship, the senior medical officers decided that all cabins should be reallocated on a basis of choice by seniority, i.e. the most senior officer had first choice, the next senior second choice, and so on. This resulted in my moving to a cabin on the starboard side, immediately aft of the Master's. He had a sweet Siamese cat and, either by choice or with the help of the Master, it was often found curled up on my bunk!

The hierarchy of medical naval officers also became very apparent at this time. The dining saloon consisted of circular tables - one of these was occupied by the senior medical officers, the next one by the remaining medical officers, and the next, a much smaller one, by the padre, supply officer, the commissioned ward master, and myself. The merchant navy officers had separate tables, and the nursing sisters dined in a separate dining room.

Apparently not many British naval ships, and certainly not a hospital ship, had docked at Port Melbourne and so we were rather a novelty. Consequently we received much publicity in the press and were also extended hospitality from public authorities and the healthcare fraternity. A few days after I joined the ship, the officers went for an all-day mini-bus drive arranged by the government publicity department. Our tour took us through the suburbs to Healesville Wildlife Sanctuary where, after lunch, we were shown various animals - cockatoos, koala bears, kangaroos, platypi, and wombats, to name just a few! It certainly brought comparative dental anatomy to life. Although the animals were in captivity, care had been taken to replicate their natural surroundings. We then proceeded to Belgravia for tea and back to Melbourne via Ferntree Gulley.

On another occasion, the Australian Red Cross escorted us on a coach tour to Dundenong and beyond, again via Ferntree Gulley, and then up a mountain range to a beautiful roadhouse at the top, the *Pig & Whistle*. Here we tucked in to a cream tea and cakes before returning to port via Croydon, Mount Albert, and Camberwell. Other visits included a conducted tour of the Royal Melbourne (New) Hospital and, a week before we left port, the maxillo-facial and plastic surgery departments of Heileburg hospital where, as in the UK, there had been many advances in techniques and provision of replacement eyes, noses, etc.

One afternoon, my Petty Officer and I were conducted over the Melbourne Dental Hospital by Dr W. J. Tuckfield who was undertaking research on the use of acrylics, acrylic dentures already being the norm in Australia. (The use of vulcanite continued in the UK and most other parts of the world as there were apparently very large stocks of rubber available after the supply from Malaya ceased following the Japanese occupation.) The hospital was a very old and dilapidated building; the erection of a new building, in the grounds of the new Royal Melbourne Hospital, had been planned but the project was postponed on the outbreak of war. There were two small surgical rooms for extractions under local anaesthesia, and an x-ray/photographic department. The dental chairs were wooden and the students had to use treadle machines, there being no electric engines available.

I was invited to the July meeting of the Victoria Branch of the Australian Dental Association, at which there were to be four speakers. The subject was children's dentistry, which was apparently a rather neglected subject in the undergraduate dental curriculum. Their association secretary, Kenneth Adamson, invited me to dinner at the Athenaeum Club before the meeting and here I met Surg./Cdr(D) Wallace RN, Surg./Cdr(D) Daniels RNVR, the Surg./Cdr(D) Royal Australian Navy (RAN), from the Flanders naval base, and Lt/Cdr(D) Rees from VA(Q).

On my first evening ashore in Melbourne I contacted the local *Everyman's Club* which resulted in an invite to a party the following Saturday evening at the house of Mrs Lucas (well renowned, I learnt later from the younger Christian fraternity, for matchmaking!) Here I met many Christian friends, including Jim Ward, who invited me to visit the university Evangelical Union (EU) annual conference with him, which was being held at *Lulla Rookh*, Tecoma the following day. I met him at Melbourne Central Station after lunch, and we proceeded by train and bus to Tecoma in time to attend the afternoon session. During the presentation, Lt. Sisly and I spoke about the IVF in the UK and opened a discussion on life in English universities in wartime. Much interest was shown and after supper we were asked to join in a general discussion with a panel of Melbourne University students on university education. At the end of the day we returned to Melbourne.

I saw Jim on various occasions and after the war he came to London for postgraduate study, obtaining not only a doctorate but also a wife! My parents and I were invited to his wedding at All Soul's, Langham Place, W1, a well-known church near Oxford Circus. On another evening, I had supper with David Angus, the prayer secretary of the EU, and he showed me various advertising material; their publicity was far in advance of that in the UK, partly due to their having a commercial advertising artist as one of their supporters.

I met the chairman of the general committee of the Crusaders Union of Victoria, Mr J.H McCracken (Jim Ward was secretary), and he explained how the movement in Australia had developed after a visit by Howard Guinness in 1929. We exchanged views on Crusader activities in our two countries. The main difference seemed to be that most Australian children attended Sunday school at their various churches and so the general rule was that Crusader bible classes did not meet on Sundays but either on a Friday or Saturday evening, or as an extra-curricular school activity in the lunch hour or after school (a school CU). I attended and spoke at several classes during our stay at Port Melbourne, and also attended meetings of their Crusader missionary fellowship, their camps committee and their senior fellowship, at which some 30 older girls and boys were present.

I was able to attend various church services in and around Melbourne; St Hilary's, Kew (C of E), Kew Baptist Church, on the anniversary of the Christian Endeavour Societies for the area, and, on our last weekend in port, Holy Trinity, Port Melbourne, for a service of prayer and thanksgiving for the Royal Navy and the Merchant Navy; the church was practically full and the Governor of Victoria attended. Our own Master, Captain A.C.M Black, MN, read one of the lessons.

We could not operate as a hospital ship during our stay in Melbourne but, when there were no interruptions to the electricity supply due to the installation of the refrigeration plant, I was able to commence dental examinations of all the ship's company to identify such treatment as would be necessary for them during the following weeks at sea.

We eventually left Port Melbourne, arriving at the entrance to Sydney harbour on 11th July and, after passing through the Sydney boom at 2030, we immediately anchored for the night. The following day, we proceeded up the harbour and tied up to a pontoon in Sirous Cove at about 1030. At 1400 I took a liberty boat to Ft Macquarie and thence to *Everyman's* where I had tea. After looking around the city in the early evening, I attended the Saturday evening social at the club. Here I again met Sub/Lt. Kennedy and also David Rogers who was now connected with the fleet newspaper department in Sydney.

The following afternoon, Sunday, I visited Sadie Philcox (nee Irwin) at her Hunters Hill home; she had been a friend of my mother's in the early 1930s when she was living in East Sheen whilst studying music in London. She received a Queensland Travelling Scholarship to study for higher music diplomas and gave several piano and vocal recitals, one at His Majesty's Theatre, before returning to Australia. Whilst she still taught music, and often acted as an accompanist at the Sydney Radio Station, she had also recently completed a course in physiotherapy, was on the staff of a local hospital and in the process of setting up her own practice.

I had lunch with the fleet dental surgeon the following week and also visited the RAN(Royal Australian Navy) stores at Glebe where, amongst other things, I was able to arrange for a cine projector and films to be delivered to the ship. One afternoon I was able to visit the Sydney Dental Hospital and was given a conducted tour by Mr Russel Boyd. It was a modern hospital, having opened in 1940 but, despite having much up-to-date equipment, was not much of an improvement on the RDH, and the students were very overcrowded. There was, however, an adequate, trained nursing staff, and a nursing sister in charge of every department. The hospital had its own in-patient department with about 16-20 beds.

We sailed from Sydney on July 18th and arrived at Manus, the BPF's anchorage in the Admiralty Islands, on July 26th after an uneventful voyage. There was little to do on the islands surrounding Manus except to bathe; the climate was very warm and sticky. We visited the main navy base on several occasions. The base dental officer was Surg./Lt (D) Martin, but apart from a small royal naval contingent, the base was all American.

Our mail was brought to this base from the UK by air, via Australia, taking less than a week in transit. It was at this time that I received two very distressing letters. The first was from my mother with news of my cousin Bill, who, being a territorial in the Honorable Artillery Company, had been called up in 1939 and served in France and Germany after the D-Day landings. He was 'mentioned in despatches'. Sadly, he had been electrocuted whilst using an electric drill to undertake DIY jobs at his home during demobilisation leave. This was very poignant for his wife Peggy, whom he married during the war, as she was pregnant with their first child. The second letter was from my dental nurse at *Collingwood* informing me of the death in Trincomalee of my fellow dental surgeon John Drury, with whom I had shared a cabin for two years.

One of the problems of being at sea for long periods in isolated parts of the world, and not being actively engaged in defeating the enemy, was loneliness, and every effort had to be made to keep up moral. One of the means to overcome this was the showing of films. Hence the reason for the Forces Film Service, of which Sir Arthur Rank was the prime supporter. The projectors were very sturdy, if somewhat noisy, and were subject to many breakdowns - all part of the fun of the show. Two of our SBAs were enthusiastic in getting to grips with the instrument and, with the help of artificers from other ships in the Fleet Train, they developed quite a good machine. Films were shared with other ships and many an afternoon was spent going from ship to ship in our launch, delivering and collecting these. We were fortunate in that our Master was a film fanatic and was always willing for one of his cadets to man the launch for this purpose. Other ships in the Fleet Train included *Baccus*, *Lancashire*, *Montclare*, *Pioneer*, and *Unicorn*.

As we were the Fleet Train hospital ship, cases were referred to us from ships both permanently at anchorage and those just visiting for a few days. After treatment, the patients who could not be returned to duty on their own ships were transferred by air to the Royal Naval Hospital in Sydney. *HMHS Vasna* paid a short visit to Manus en route from New Zealand to India and so I was able to chat with Vic Simons. We had dinner together on each other's ships.

There was great excitement on 6th August when, at 0115, the alarm was sounded for a fire in number two hold. With prompt action from surrounding ships, and the aid of their fire-fighting equipment, the hold was flooded and the fire extinguished within twelve hours. There was moderate damage to stores, nearly all Red Cross stores being lost, and other damage by flooding to many areas of the ship. There was 18 inches of water in the dental department which caused damage to some stores. The electric engine and vulcaniser burnt out, but were repaired by Fleet Train personnel within 14 days to a better standard than previously. Most of the damaged stores were replaced by *Montclare*, although the specialist dental stores had to be sent from Sydney.

As soon as hostilities with Japan ceased, following the dropping of atom bombs on Hiroshima and Nagasaki, the Fleet Train gradually dispersed to other locations, mainly Hong Kong. This was to be our next destination. We set sail on September 2nd, arriving in

Hong Kong, where there was still some firing to be heard in the hills above the harbour, on the 13th.

By the time we arrived in Hong Kong, most of the Fleet Train was already there. At anchor were many Royal Navy ships including *Anson*, *Duke of York*, *Queensborough*, *Pioneer* and *Venerable*. *Sir Bruce Fraser* arrived on 14th September. We did not remain in Hong Kong for long and at dawn on 16th September we set sail for Hainan Island under the escort of the destroyer *Kepenfeld*. Our mission was to embark prisoners of war (POW) and convey them to Manilla where the *HMNZHS Maunganui* would be waiting to convey any Australians to their homeland.

We arrived in Suma Bay at dawn where we immediately anchored, our escort having reported mines in the area. We commenced embarking about 140 POWs at 09.30, both walking and stretcher cases being brought alongside by landing craft, completing the operation by 1100. They had received no Red Cross parcels and very few medical supplies in over three years of captivity and were all very excited about coming onto our beautiful ship. The story told by our padre in a radio broadcast in Perth a few months later best describes the stamina and moral of these men:

> The men were weak and badly starved, but their mental outlook was unbelievably cheerful. The senior officer of the survivors was an Australian Army captain. He did not know much about the navy, but he had heard something about saluting the quarter deck. Although unsteady on his feet, he dragged himself to the top of the gangway and tried to salute, but he could not make it - it was one of the most pathetic things I had ever seen.

We sailed again at noon, bound for Manilla, but when we were *en route* we received a signal instructing us to return directly to Hong Kong, where we arrived on the 23rd. Strangely, no one had knowledge of any counter-instructions having been sent to us and such was the level of concern when we did not arrive in Manilla as planned that the American navy had been searching for us in the approaches to Manilla! There was much confusion in these early post-war days!

As well as attending to their medical needs, the staff entertained the POWs as much as possible and we were able to provide film shows each evening on the open deck. The Australian POW walking cases, together with many other military personnel, were eventually accommodated in the hangers of the small 'lend-lease' aircraft carriers that were returning to Australia. The stretcher cases remained with us and the seriously ill were evacuated to Australia by air. There was only one death on board, a young Australian, and the padre and I, together with two of his fellow ex-prisoners, were able to visit his grave (10221, sector 17b) and take photographs that our padre enclosed in a letter to the young man's parents.

Our duties in Hong Kong were basically to act as base hospital until St Mary's Hospital was operational again after the occupation; we were kept quite busy. At one stage, the ship was placed in quarantine for a week owing to a case of smallpox. We lay at anchor close to Lei U Mun peninsular, from where recreational parties could easily go ashore during off-duty periods. One day some of us climbed up the highest peak (Tim-U-Tai 950 ft) from where we had a good view of Hong Kong, all of the surrounding British Territory, and part of mainland China itself. We passed a Chinese Temple and several Chinese graves on the climb and saw bodies of children that had been washed up on the seashore.

Our padre was sick himself for a period and I substituted for him, taking several parties ashore. One Sunday I conducted the broadcast parade service for him as none of the other officers were interested.

On these various onshore excursions, we had the opportunity to drive around the island in either Royal Marine transport or vehicles loaned to us by other services. Places we visited included the cathedral, Stanley Camp, St Mary's Hospital, Deepwater Bay and Happy Valley. The local Roman Catholic chaplain asked us to undertake a dental inspection of the nuns at the local convent. Despite their having no dental treatment available for several years, their dental condition was remarkably good and only five required extractions.

HMHS Oxfordshire arrived from the north with many ex-prisoners of war and ex-interned civilians of various nationalities. It had apparently been agreed that we should convey those heading south to Australia on their homeward journey. From Hong Kong, the *Oxfordshire* was to proceed to the UK with British personnel and also disembark any other nationals *en route*. One day they invited us to a cocktail party on board when the Commander in Chief, Commodore, Hong Kong and others were present. We proceeded alongside at Kowloon Jetty on 15th November, embarked further civilian passengers who had been interned in China for the duration of the war, and eventually sailed for Australia on November 17th.

A few days out, when we were beginning to formalise a programme of events for our passengers, a 12-year-old girl, Elizabeth Edwards, spotted the Crusader badge that was attached to my identification bracelet. She had been at the CIM school at Cheefoo where there had been a Crusader class. I learnt from her that there were some 18 missionary families on board and that her own mother had died in captivity. Elizabeth has contacted me since then and I know that she returned to China with her father after the war, eventually going on to study at Melbourne University and later taking a theological course. When I heard from her in 1986 she was the married mother of four children, three at university and the youngest still at school.

All our staff did their very best not only to provide for the medical needs of our passengers and entertaining them, but also to help them in any others ways that they could. On our arrival in Fremantle, a letter was received extending grateful thanks to everyone for care and attention received on the voyage. It read, 'This is not merely a conventional expression of thanks, but a sincere appreciation. Your care of the sick and entertainment of the children, constant care for the welfare of all the passengers, tended to make the voyage a most enjoyable and memorable one.'

After spending the night at anchor in Gage Roads, Fremantle, we docked at number eight berth, North Wharf, at 0900 on Saturday 3rd December. Whilst arrangements had been made for CIM and CMS personnel by their respective societies, we found that no arrangements had been made for the accommodation and onward transportation of service personnel. This was particularly distressing for the families of several very sick patients who had to remain on board for some days before they could be discharged ashore.

The chaplain and I had a busy time ashore contacting naval authorities in Fremantle, the welfare officer at Leurwin, and the Phyllis Dean Hostel, in order to make arrangements for shore holiday leave for sick berth staff. We were fortunate in meeting Mr Bishop, a manager of *Shell Mex*, who drove us around Perth in the afternoon thus enabling us to obtain a list of leave addresses and contact Regional Transport Offices about travelling facilities. Mr Bishop also introduced us to the Australian Comforts Fund and the British Red Cross resulting in a considerable quantity of Comforts and games equipment being delivered on board before we left port. In the evening, we visited the Missions to Seamen in Fremantle and met Rev Heerdigan and Rev Watt. The following day, we returned to Perth to finalize the leave arrangements and obtain travel warrants, etc.

During our time in Western Australia I was able to renew contacts with Crusaders and IVF, meeting Jim Ward again and also Major Murray Clarke of the Hollywood Hospital who was a member of the IVF Australian Central Council. I attended a graduate's fellowship reunion at which he was the speaker.

Our padre, Rev Janes, and I spent seven days leave with the Bishop of Bunbury and his wife, Bishop and Mrs Knight, travelling overnight on December 10th and returning by afternoon train on the 17th. He had a diocese larger than the whole of England and Wales and Mrs Knight was the president of the MU for the whole of Australia. I think Mrs Knight must have written to my mother when she learnt of her interest in the MU as they visited us when they were in the UK for the next Lambeth Conference. My mother and she corresponded for the rest of their lives. We sailed from Fremantle for Singapore at 0900 on December 23rd.

On Christmas Eve we celebrated communion at midnight, a service which included the singing of carols. There was also a service of carols and bible readings on Christmas Day morning, after which we distributed parcels which had been given to us by the Missions to Seamen, around the ship. The officers were 'at home' to the chief and petty officers before lunch and we visited the junior mess in the evening after dinner. We also had a midnight service on New Year's Eve.

We only had a few passengers on board and the relationship between crew and passengers was in distinct contrast to that on the journey south. The passengers were mainly men who were returning to their Malaysian businesses or plantations following the cessation of hostilities and, as a privilege, the government had offered them free passage on our ship to get them there as quickly as possible. They took the attitude that they should be treated as first class passengers and started ordering everyone around with the result that......!

It was on January 2nd that we arrived in Singapore and nobody really seemed to be expecting us. I went ashore the following day and managed to contact the Fleet Dental Officer, the Fleet Film Officer, etc. The place seemed to be in a state of organized chaos! Eventually we took on the duties of base hospital whilst facilities ashore were being brought up to pre-war standards. One day I bumped into Captain Geoffrey Baker, Royal Army Service Corps, one of the VPS camps officers I had met in Stamford in 1941. His unit had been fighting their way from India. He told me that my cousin, Dick Wootton, who was by this time a Red Cross commissioner, was in the area, but I never met up with him. Geoff came aboard for dinner one evening.

One Sunday we were able to attend evensong at the cathedral and we heard the Bishop of Colombo preach. We also went to the communion service on Easter Sunday morning. The church was packed, with some members of the congregation standing in the aisles and choir area. Others stood around the outside of the church.

We went ashore quite often and were able to purchase pineapples and bananas. I also bought some cigars for my father. One day we collected a three-ton army truck at Clifford Pier and took a party of ship's personnel across the island and causeway into Jehore and then north eastwards to Kota Tinggi, stopping for a picnic in a rubber plantation on the way. We then went on to some waterfalls where we were able to bathe, followed by an exploration of the surrounding territory. It was 1830 before we eventually arrived back at Clifford Pier.

On 11th March we went alongside and discharged all our patients to shore hospitals and then went out into the roads about three miles from Clifford Pier to await 'further instructions'.

* * * * *

The war being over, a system of demobilisation was promulgated by the Admiralty. Various factors were taken into account in deciding the order of discharge of personnel, including age and duration of service. This resulted in a gradual changeover of staff as people left for the UK. Only some of them were replaced. My dental Petty Officer was soon on his way back to civvy street and one of the SBAs, George 'Chippy' Carpenter, took over his duties.

On the 24th April it was my turn and I joined the troopship SS *Orantes* for passage to the UK. Although all the 32 bunks in our large cabin were occupied by naval personnel, the greater number of officers on board were either army or air force. There was no dental surgery but an army emergency kit was available in the troop hospital, although cooperation with medical staff was difficult. On board the ship there was a library but it had rather a poor selection of books and so card games or Monopoly became our main pastimes after dark. One of the Fleet Air Officers, with whom we played Monopoly, sadly developed a mental disorder and eventually had to be restrained in the hospital. He was discharged ashore at Port Said and, we learnt later, was flown back to the UK for treatment.

We docked at Southampton on 16th May 1946, where I was met by my father. I passed through customs with minimum of delay and then took the train to London. My father was working in the city by this time, the Kirkby establishment having closed (no further bombs were required!), and so I travelled on the afternoon train to Liverpool alone and then onward to Kirkby to see my mother who had remained there until other accommodation was available in the south. At the end of my leave I had to return to the Admiralty in London for routine debriefing.

Whilst I was in Singapore, I had received a letter from Norman Gray, a dental surgeon in Eastbourne, inquiring whether I might be interested in joining his practice as an assistant; my name had been given to him by Douglas Johnson, the then general secretary of the IVF. I went for an interview with him in June and joined him in his practice in July. Also during June, I saw Professor H. Stobie at the RDH in London and he offered me the post of Demonstrator in the Parodontal Department. It was for two half-days per week as from September and I accepted.

Although I was now a civilian again I was still, of course, on the reserve list and whilst I was in Eastbourne, I applied to transfer to the permanent RNVR. The various Divisions had not been reorganised following the cessation of hostilities and the Sussex Division was full. However, shortly after I moved to London in 1948/9, I was invited for interview on *HMS President* (the London headquarters of the RNVR) moored on the River Thames, and I was granted a permanent commission. This committed me to attending at the surgery on board the sister ship, *HMS Chrysanthemum*, moored astern of her, about once a month, attending the annual inspection in the summer each year, and a fortnight training period at a Royal Navy shore establishment or on a ship every two years (for which I received normal naval pay and privileges). I attended various courses at the Naval Medical School, Alverstoke, and the maxillo-facial centre at Park Prewett Hospital, Basingstoke.

My first appointment was to an aircraft carrier that was being used for the sea training of cadets and lay at anchor in Portland Harbour. There was also a week's intensive drill at the naval base at Portsmouth, in preparation for the RNVR victory parade and inspection by HM The Queen on the Horse Guards Parade, London. For this we were accommodated in one of the forts on the hills behind Portsmouth. This was followed by a week at Royal Marine Barracks, Deal.

Other training was spent at the naval air bases at Culdrose and Lossiemouth and *HMS Cochrane* for duties at HM Dockyard, Rosyth. For one training period I was based at a naval establishment in Germany on the Rhine and was able to visit various other military and air force bases whilst there. I also remember being on a ship on Gareloch, in the Firth of Clyde (a few miles north of Helensburgh) when they were frantically preparing laid up naval ships for sea when the Suez crisis was imminent.

When I had completed the required time of service, I was promoted to Surgeon Lieutenant Commanded (D), and was eventually awarded the Volunteer Reserve Decoration.

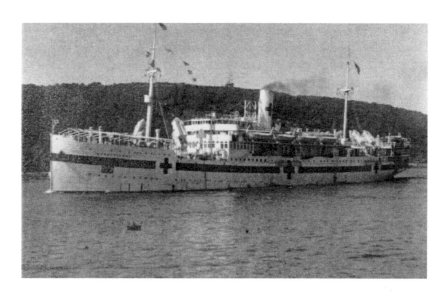

HMHS Gerusalemme

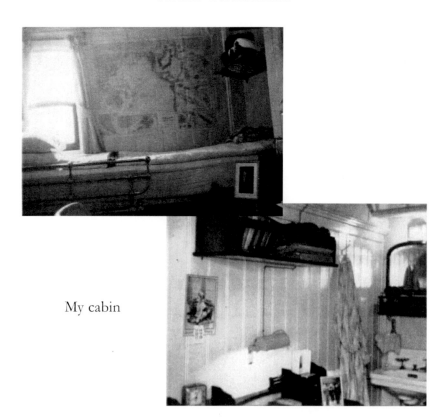

My cabin

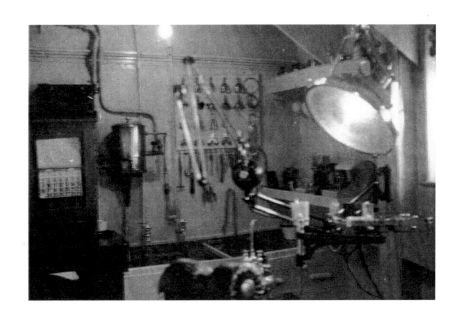

Dental surgery on board

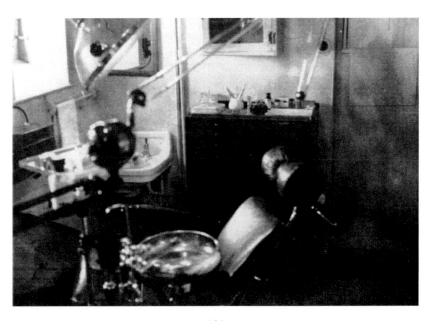

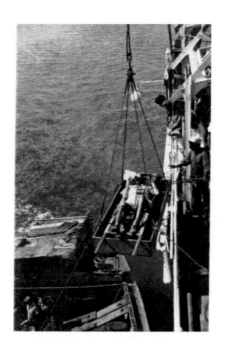

Evacuation stretcher case POW's from Hainan Island

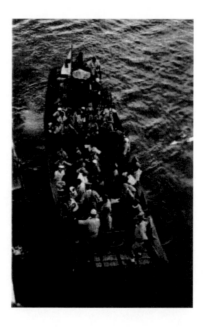

Non-stretcher cases being evacuated

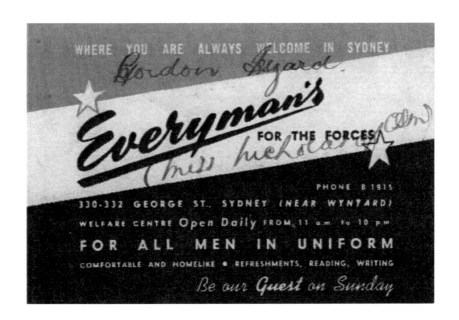

Everyman's Club in Sydney, Australia

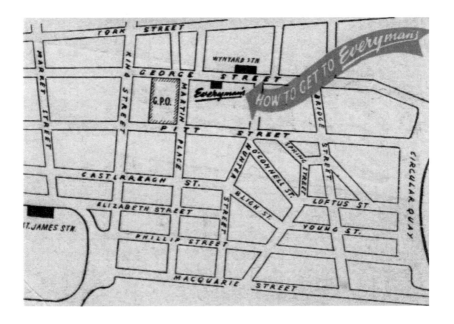

Learning Curves

Between the time of my interview and my arrival in Eastbourne, Mr Gray had kindly arranged full-board accommodation for me with an elderly member of the congregation of Holy Trinity Church who lived in Upperton Road. This proved to be in a very convenient situation close to the centre of the town, and every Sunday morning I rode with this lady in her taxi to church! It was understood that this was to be temporary accommodation and I eventually moved to Enys Road, where my new landlady was a member of the Visick family who had formerly owned the dental practice with Mr Gray.

The original practice in College Road had been partially destroyed by a bomb and, with Mr Visick having retired to Cheltenham during the war, Mr Gray purchased a new three-storey building, number 16, almost opposite the old practice. The building, a large double-fronted structure, mid-way between the town centre and the sea front, was converted so that the practice occupied the ground floor. On the first and second floors were two flats, with separate entrances. A waiting room and large surgery occupied the front of the building and there was a further large surgery at the rear (where Mr Gray operated). I had a small surgery in-between.

It was very difficult to find dental surgery equipment following the war, and we could only obtain sufficient to equip and use the rear surgery and my surgery. Mr Gray transferred his equipment from his home, where he'd had his main practice during the war, and mine came from his small branch surgery a few miles inland, from where he had operated during the time when the town was suffering constant 'hit and run' raids. Fortunately, a relation of Hubert Visick, a garage owner in Eastbourne, was a very good engineer and installed various modern surgery accessories which made us the envy of many local dental surgeons. There was also a small office at the practice which was occupied by the secretary, Miss Wybrow, and a large laboratory for our dental technician, Mr Dodd, and his assistants.

It is of interest to note that when we rummaged through the bombed contents of the old Visick/Gray practice, we found a large number of glass lantern slides depicting many types of removable orthodontic appliances that were used in the pre-war years. I think these were donated either to the BDA museum or that of the British Society for the Study of Orthodontics (BSSO). Mr Visick had not only been a much respected orthodontist, but also a keen amateur photographer.

Mr Gray was absent from the practice on a couple of occasions. The first was for the Gray family holiday in late July, the second, when he led the Eastbourne Crusaders on a Broads sailing holiday in August. This latter excursion was the revival of a tradition of sailing holidays which had been popular before the war. (Mr Gray was a keen yachtsman, a member of the Eastbourne Sailing Club, and also owned his own boat. He was affectionately known as 'The Admiral'.) The result was that I was left in charge of the practice to deal with emergency cases, there being very few other patients who were prepared to be treated by a recently demobilised forces dental surgeon! My other challenge with regard to securing patients was that Mr Gray's wife, and her mother, kept a very tight control on the clientele of the practice.

Mr Gray was a well respected dental surgeon and businessman in the town. Between the two wars he had studied at the Angle Orthodontic School in the USA and had also obtained an Edinburgh Higher Dental Diploma qualification. In the 1950s he was awarded an honorary Fellowship in Dental Surgery and a Diploma in Orthodontics. He was the immediate past president of the BSSO and a respected member of the European Orthodontic Society. I used to attend with him the monthly meetings of the BSSO in London and was eventually admitted as a member of the society.

In addition to his large orthodontic practice, Mr Gray was honorary dental surgeon to local hospitals and orthodontist to the school dental service. There were also many boarding schools in and around Eastbourne and many of the pupils went to him for orthodontic treatment. Most of this treatment was with removable appliances (Mr Dodd being a very skilled dental technician), but some fixed appliances were constructed using gold attachments and wires. Stainless steel bands and 'archwires' were just being introduced and one of the new Watkin portable dental welders had been installed in the practice.

* * * * *

It was not long before I was once again involved with Crusaders. Having served as an assistant leader at the Banstead class before I joined the Royal Navy, I was naturally invited to attend and help with the running of this class, attending leaders' meetings and the like. Our leaders were Norman Gray, Willie Prentice (an assistant bank manager) and Dr Snowball (a retired CIM missionary). I became the first secretary of the Sussex Area Committee (Brighton, Eastbourne, Lewes, Seaford, and Worthing) and we held our first weekend conference at the recently purchased Crusader Westbrook Centre on the Isle of Wight, an estate that was dedicated as a memorial to those Crusaders who had paid the supreme sacrifice during World War II.

For many years prior to the war, it had been a class tradition to organise an annual class sailing cruise on the Norfolk Broads and, as already mentioned, these were now revived. During the absence of the sailing group, I chaired the weekly Sunday afternoon Crusader class meetings. When the sailors returned from their trips, they brought back considerable footage of 16mm film, taken by senior members, and we had great fun in editing this to show at parent gatherings and the like. The floor would be strewn with sections of the film and fun had by all in organising it in the right sections. The same process occurred after Mr Gray filmed David Tryon's Anglesey Pioneer camps in 1948.

I continued to travel to Holy Trinity Church in the shared taxi until my bicycle arrived from Kirkby, although I usually walked home with friends. Within a few weeks of my arrival, the vicar, Canon S.M. Warner, asked me if I would take over the leadership of the

Campaigners. I discovered that this was not a branch of the youth organisation of the same name, but a group of people from various denominations in the town (of about the same age as myself), who had banded together during the war years. They met each week for prayer and fellowship and conducted various Christian activities in the locality. This proved to be a very worthwhile organisation which welded the various denominations together, and was the means of introducing some members to full-time Christian service.

Over the years, the group had a great impact on many Christian activities in the town. One of these was the organisation of an open air meeting on the promenade. This took place on a Sunday evening after the church service during the summer months. In September, lantern talks (using a lantern with electrodes producing an arc light, and 3.5 inch glass slides) were given by Canon Warner at the Old Lifeboat Station, the pictures being projected onto the wall of the building. These meetings drew a large crowd of residents and visitors to hear a simple gospel message.

At Holy Trinity's annual parochial meeting, I was elected to the PCC. I also became a sidesman, being given responsibility for certain gated pews. Most of the pews were 'rented' by parishioners - an ancient custom that was quite common in churches at this time and which provided them with a guaranteed income. These pews were reserved for them to within five minutes of the commencement of services and part of my role was to oversee this. I also read at least one of the lessons at morning and evening services. There were no microphones in those days and so clarity was important, especially with an elderly congregation with hearing difficulties (their old type hearing aids whistled if they increased the volume because they could not hear you!)

Once a month the Sunday afternoon Sunday school, a thriving organisation with nearly 100 pupils, had a service in church. The curate used to conduct this but when he was not replaced during the war years, Canon Warner assumed this role. As he was now elderly and not in good health, he asked me if I would do it for him.

Shortly after my arrival in the town, Ross Tully joined our congregation. He had just been demobilised following service with the Gurkha regiment and had moved to Eastbourne with his family. He had been accepted for ordination training and was waiting for a vacancy at a training college. Ross helped with both these monthly services, reading the lessons on some Sundays, and in many other ways within the church. He was eventually accepted at Ridley Hall in Cambridge. I spent several weekends there with him and we became life-long friends.

Canon Warner died suddenly in 1947, two days after Christmas, his series of sermons during Advent having been on the 'second coming'. Shortly after his death, the churchwardens invited Ross and me into Canon Warner's study to choose some books to keep in remembrance of him. We both chose one of his bibles (I have mine to this day) and, amongst other tomes, Ross choose books that would help him in his studies for the ministry and I selected several of the bound copies of *Living Water*, a monthly periodical that Canon Warner used to edit on behalf of his fellow Keswick Convention trustees.

As a result of Canon Warner's sudden death, there was a very long interregnum, during which period the churchwardens conducted the services. A dear elderly gentleman (over 80 years old), a life-long friend of Canon Warner who had been on the staff of the London City Mission for many years, travelled down from London each weekend officiating at Communion services and often preaching.

As a memorial to their vicar and friend of so many years, the parishioners replaced one of the plain glass windows with a stained glass window of Holman Hunt's 'The Light of the World', and the Campaigners presented a framed portrait of Canon Warner which was hung in the vestry with those of other past incumbents of the church.

One of the good things that arose following the comradeship that developed between Christians in the armed forces of both our own country and those of the USA, was the organisation Youth For Christ (YFC). As far as is known, Eastbourne was one of the first towns in the UK where regular monthly YFC meetings were held. Following a visit from one of their representatives, a committee of local church members was formed under the chairmanship of Willie Prentice, and the demonstration theatre of the gas showrooms in Terminus Road was booked for a series of monthly Saturday evening rallies. Willie Prentice was a very versatile pianist and, with the help of homemade glass slides and the same projector as we used for the autumn open air services (35mm projectors were not then on the market), the words of the new American choruses were projected onto a screen. This method is now used in many churches today, but with much more sophisticated optics than were available to us. Thus, a type of rally entirely new to our generation was born.

Another first were the well produced invitations and posters (both in glorious technicolour) that a local Christian printer produced using the latest state of the art printing techniques. The posters were not only displayed on church noticeboards, but also at local railway stations and on buses. As publicity secretary, I was responsible for this part of the organisation. The rallies were made as attractive as possible, with the aim of presenting the gospel of Christ to the youth of our land. We had the help of many guest speakers and these rallies continued long after I left the area. Eventually, the UK headquarters of YFC was established in Eastbourne and I discovered in later years that a senior Crusader, who during the early part of the war had helped me with the junior section of Banstead Crusaders, had become a member of the YFC staff.

* * * * *

What of our family during my stay in Eastbourne? When I first arrived, my mother, with all our furniture, was still at our wartime farmhouse in Kirkby. My father who, as explained in a previous chapter, had been moved to London with the MoS and was responsible for disposing surplus wartime equipment, was living with my grandmother in a very small bungalow at Bexleyheath, Kent. Accommodation in Eastbourne, as elsewhere in the country, was very scarce, with many demobilised personnel needing homes. Eventually we found a small top floor flat in a converted building in Blackwater Road and, whilst we were waiting for the building works to be completed, my mother and father (and Taffy) stayed on full-board terms in a guest house in the town. When the building work was complete we were able to move into our new home and for the first time in nine years, we were all together again.

At this time, food, clothing, and petrol were still in short supply and rigorous rationing restrictions were in force. Our car, which my mother had purchased second-hand in 1937 (it was then nearly 10 years old) had served us well, especially during the war years, but was now beginning to show its age, and most spares were unobtainable. Unfortunately it broke down near Horley, Sussex, when we were on our way to John Ruff's wedding. The AA could only make temporary repairs and it was at this point that we decided it was best to sell it. I, as a dental surgeon, although not eligible to purchase a new car, could register with a garage for a second-hand post-war car when one became available. This I did, but we had moved from Eastbourne before one became available and I had to travel back to collect it.

It gradually became obvious that my joining Mr Gray's practice was not working out as he had envisaged. He had the idea that I should be introducing new patients to the practice but I never did understand how I was meant to achieve this as I was unknown in the town. Also, the friends I made were patients of other practices where fees were considerably less than ours (these were the days before the NHS), and many of them belonged to Friendly Societies who helped with the cost of dental treatment through the 'dental letter' system, which was not acceptable to Mr Gray. It gradually became clear that I would need to move on.

It was an unfortunate situation but overall I did gain from the experience, and I certainly treated some interesting patients. I well remember providing new full upper and lower dentures for one retired missionary (all missionaries received free treatment), the grandson of the founder of the CIM. He was a lovely 90-year-old gentleman with a flowing white beard who was living with his daughter-in-law in the town. What fun taking upper and lower plaster impressions (modern impression materials were not yet available in this country), and the beard!!!

I was not without a job, however, as Mr Vernon Thurston, whose wife had encouraged me to enter the profession whilst I was still at school, had written to me shortly after I left the navy, imploring me to help him out at his practice in the City of London. As he was still without any assistance, I was able to become his part-time assistant, travelling to London daily. I also increased my sessions at the RDH, the salaries of dental school staff having recently been increased to what one could earn in general practice.

Mr Thurston had a busy practice, catering mainly for those employed in the city, many of whom could only attend either during their lunch hour or after work. They were consequently very pleased when I was able to provide a few evening sessions after we moved to Cockfosters. Before the introduction of the NHS in 1948, many of the patients, particularly junior staff of city firms, could only afford treatment when they had a 'dental letter' from their Friendly Society, who then paid a proportion of fees (a common facility in those days).

I stayed with Mr Thurston until I was appointed as half-time senior dental registrar at St George's Hospital, Hyde Park Corner. This appointment dovetailed very conveniently with my half-time appointment at the Royal, to the benefit of all parties, especially as these two hospitals later formed a teaching group.

The Dental Scene

I sometimes feel that those of our colleagues who commenced their professional training after the Second World War, and more so those who joined the profession in the 1960s and after, fail to appreciate the difficulties that we had in putting the 'blood and vulcanite' era behind us. It was a huge task to re-educate the public (and in some instances our older professional colleagues) in the advances that had been made in techniques, and to persuade them that the health of the whole mouth was just as important as that of the whole body, and that extractions were not the only answer to dental pain. This situation was not helped by the fact that the old syllabus, as laid down in the 1921 Dentist Act, which required students to construct a set number of full upper and lower dentures (from impression stage to final fitting) during their first two years at dental school, remained.

The so-called 'gas sessions' (using foot controlled nitrous oxide/air anaesthetic apparatus) in hospital out-patients and school dental clinics were commonplace for at least a further two decades. Although anaesthetic procedures have improved, such procedures were often a child's first experience of dentistry. Many were traumatised for life by the experience and, as a result, never had any regular dental care until a clearance and dentures became necessary. The lesson of 'prevention is better than cure' had still to be learnt.

Professor F. C. Wilkinson, Dean of Manchester Dental School, in his forward to *An Investigation and Recommendations concerning the Future of Dentistry*, a report by the JPCDS (representing all the UK dental schools) in 1942, highlights this situation when, after stressing the difficult task that confronts the authors, continues, 'They inherit a profession drained dry by the price paid for the 1921 Act, but at a stage presenting greater opportunities for inspired leadership than at any previous time. Their immediate concern has wisely been with education, not only because it is an aspect of dentistry they can approach with knowledge at least as profound as that of most of their elders, but because it is the foundation upon which the progress and development of the profession must be built.' Many of the advances in the profession suggested by future post-war planners incorporated both the recommendations made in this report and in future reports of the JPCDS. At least two of the dental students who were involved in this became deans of dental schools, and several later held high offices in the profession.

Those of us who served in the forces during the Second World War saw first-hand the poor dental health of recruits, more so those of us appointed to initial reception units, and we did our best to provide some dental oral hygiene education. However, it was probably the introduction of new materials, new techniques, and the improved education of the dental student that eventually, after many years, gradually resulted in the improvements we find today.

When I was senior hospital dental officer at Highlands Hospital, North London, I can well remember the experiments being made by the late Paul Toller, and others, with high speed drills, using cylinders of compressed air. Acrylics were replacing rubber (vulcanite) as a denture base and for some filling materials. Due to the high breakage rate of dentures of post-encephalitis lethurgica patients, we undertook a research project using nylon as a denture base material; however with the advance in stainless steel casting techniques, this became a more preferable material.

Whilst on the junior teaching staff of the RDH, I became a member of the Junior Staff Committee. This put me in an ideal position, along with my colleagues, to improve those elements we had found lacking in our own student days. We had all been in the dental branch of one of the armed forces and had seen for ourselves not only the poor dental health of personnel, but also the inadequate treatment they had received before and after being 'called-up'. How could we improve this and the overall dental curriculum? It seemed a daunting task. Students had to be taught to view the mouth as an integral part of the whole human body. They needed to see their role as not just to repair it when that was necessary, but to ensure the lasting improvements that new techniques could provide, thus promoting not only the overall health of the mouth, but also that of the body as a whole.

A new photographic department, with an excellent, well qualified photographer, had now been established at the Royal and, with the advancements in colour photograph (35mm slides and 16mm film), we were able to produce slides and films to use as teaching-aids. I used these to speak on my speciality, gingivectomy, at BDA meetings all around London. Also, the junior staff mounted a joint demonstration at a BDA annual conference in Newcastle on 'The aetiology of mal-occlusion', showing the importance of treating the mouth as a whole and each individual tooth as part of an intricate dentition.

The training of Dental Hygienists was another area that had needed to be addressed. Advancements here led to a vast improvement in general dental health. The Royal Air Force had instituted its own programme of training, and their Dental Hygienists were allowed to treat their personnel in clinics where a dental officer was present. It wasn't until the late '40s that legislation on training was incorporated into the Dental Act, at which time a training scheme for Dental Hygienists was established at the Eastman Dental Hospital. Those who completed the two year approved course, with examinations, were then allowed to undertake certain clinical procedures under the care of a qualified dental surgeon. This scheme was a great success and was a definite step forward in dental health education.

The introduction of the National Health Service in 1948 caused many problems. The dental profession had fought hard for dental hospital staff to hold the same grades and conditions of service as those of their medical colleagues, but even this produced problems. I was at that time employed part-time in the dental department of St George's Hospital, Hyde Park Corner, as a senior dental officer. The Governor came down to the dental department to say that as I was too young to be employed at that grade and would I be happy to accept the grade of Senior Registrar, there being little difference in the rates of pay. This proved very important to me in my future career and also established this training grade in the future dental structure of this teaching hospital. At the same time, it did produce other problems as there were no dental house surgeon grades at this hospital, nor at most other general hospitals at this time, and such appointments were necessary if a training path was to be established. It was not long before a House Surgeon was appointed at St George's but it remained a national problem for many years to come. My paper entitled, *Dental House Surgeons to be or not to be*, read as my inaugural address as chairman of the North West Metropolitan Hospitals Group of the BDA in 1956, shows how very little had been achieved to overcome this problem.

These were exciting times following the many horrors and traumas of six years of war, and the profession was only just beginning to realise its many future opportunities. Meetings had had to be curtailed or cancelled altogether during these years and were only now beginning to revive their previous schedules. Several new societies were established as a result of wartime experiences and the war also precipitated the development of new techniques and the discovery of new drugs and materials.

In 1949 a number of us who were interested in periodontology met together at the Eastman Dental Hospital, resulting in the inaugural meeting, on the 19th July, of the British Society of Periodontology, myself being a founder member. As a result of these activities, I made many professional acquaintances, friendships which lasted many years. A scheme was started soon after the end of the war whereby professionals from America organised courses in various parts of the world, in subjects that due to wartime restrictions, their colleagues had been unable to read up about in Papers and Journals, thus denying them the opportunity to assimilate advancing knowledge and learn recent techniques. The Royal arranged for me to attend one of these courses, on the subject of periodontology, which took place in Utrect, Holland, in 1948.

It was also in this period that the Christian Dental Fellowship (CDF) was formed. Shortly after I moved from Eastbourne to Cockfosters, Dr Douglas Johnson (who was then general secretary of the IVF), invited me to join the committee of the Graduates Fellowship of that organisation, who were in turn anxious that a dental section of this branch of the organisation be formed. Consequently, at a meeting of a few dental members following the Graduates Fellowship reunion on Saturday 16th September 1950, a dental group indeed was formed. Shortly afterwards, Douglas Johnson wrote, 'Don't be too disappointed with a small start; remember the Church only had one great "Man" plus eleven trembling disciples at the start - it is the one who turns the scales.' How true these words have proved to be, for it is only through the power of God that the CDF has grown to the size it is today.

For the next 15+ years I acted as secretary/organiser of this new group and although there was always a President and Treasurer, it was not until the mid 1960's that officers such as General Secretary, Missionary, Secretary, Conference Secretary, Students Liaison Officer were elected, and later an editor of the very successful 'Newsround' was appointed. During these years we registered as a 'charity' and for many years I was responsible for organising Covenanted Giving that was later superseded by Gift Aid. I was elected President for four years and at the Golden Jubilee Celebrations had the honour of President Emerirus bestowed upon me.

With a small membership, scattered as it was throughout the United Kingdom, the logistics of arranging meetings of members was always a problem. This was partly overcome by arranging annual conferences, the first of which was at Old Jordan's, Beaconsfield, Buckinghamshire, with just 16 present. We then moved to Mabledon, Tonbridge, Kent, for several years, and then to various other parts of the country - Weston-super-mare, Hiltenborough in Kent, Edinburgh, Eastbourne, Ashburnham in Sussex, Torquay, Harrogate, Bournemouth, Ross-on-Wye, Llanfairfechan, and Herne Bay, to name just a few.

Gradually these developed into family conferences (the CDF led the way in this type of conference) with a special, separate programme for children. It has to be said that the outreach to the dental profession was much greater in those early days than it is today.

When the 11th International Dental Congress was held at the Royal Festival Hall in July 1952, the CDF arranged a reception for delegates in Church House, Westminster. Over 120 delegates from 19 different countries attended and the film *Hidden Treasurers* was shown, introduced by Norman Gray, who was at that time secretary of the European Orthodontic Society, later to become the first President of CDF.

We enjoyed close liaison with the BDA and each autumn, we arranged a meeting for all those connected with the profession at their headquarters (both when they were at Hill Street and when they moved to Wimpole Street), and news of our activities regularly appeared in their journal. We also regularly had a stand at their annual conference where we arranged a missionary breakfast or tea.

During the early years, we commenced courses on emergency dentistry for non-dental missionary candidates and missionaries home on furlough, with the aim of instructing them in simple dental procedures they could carry out in the field. These included lectures on basic dental health, which we hoped would be of help to them when they were in isolated locations overseas (travel for treatment not being so easy or sophisticated as it is today!) These courses were presented at, amongst other places, Birkenhead, Birmingham, Chislehurst, Edinburgh, Glasgow, Taplow, and central London.

As members of the Graduate Fellowship, we also joined with other sections of the organisation in the annual exhibition in North London for missionaries. Each section had a stand depicting how they may be able to assist the missionaries by providing material or supplies for their various needs.

We all appreciate that times have changed and some of the services that the CDF have provided in the past are no longer needed, but the primary object of the Fellowship, that of outreach to the profession, seems to have been neglected, with preference being given to sending members overseas to provide Christian teaching and dental treatment to those of other countries. Does it need to amend its ways?

Another organisation with which I became involved, especially after we moved to Surrey in 1971, was The Churches Council for Health and Healing, in which there were representatives of many mainstream churches, from the various medical professions and from other organisations with health care as their central concern. It was chaired by the Right Reverend Morris Maddocks, who had recently resigned from his appointment as Bishop of Selby where he was also the advisor to the Archbishops of both Canterbury and York on the ministry of health and healing. In his ministry he regularly stressed his belief in the healing of the whole body (body, mind, and spirit) and the healing power of listening. I represented both the CDF and the British Dental Association. Through this organisation I had opportunity to meet with many people of like beliefs to my own and to discuss with them a wide range of different topics. I regularly submitted reports to the British Dental Journal (BDJ).

There had been a Guild of Health since 1904 and this new organisation was complementary to it, their outreach extending to many churches throughout our country and overseas. It is a tribute to their perseverance that this outreach continues to this day.

More Opportunities

One of the challenges of moving to London was finding living accommodation. With the great destruction of property during the bombing raids, and the large number of ex-service personnel needing somewhere in the city to live, the housing situation was much more acute than it had been in Eastbourne. I was fortunate, however, for I received a phone call from Raymond Bird (a fellow student from the Royal who was working as a stipendiary dental officer at the RDH whilst building up his practice in Waltham Cross), telling me that a small flat was becoming vacant in the block where he lived. Would we be interested? We certainly were and, despite it being very cramped accommodation for us, we accepted - 'beggars can't be choosers'.

So that's how we came to live in Cockfosters. The area was very convenient for both my father and I to travel into the City. It also suited my mother, as it meant she could catch up with her pre-war friends. We soon became very involved in local church activities, my mother joining the choir and supporting the MU, eventually becoming one of the diocesan speakers for the Diocese of London. I became a sidesman again and, at the next annual general meeting (AGM), was elected as a member of the PCC.

Professionally, I continued with my teaching appointment on the staff of the RDH and developed the periodontal department. Details of developments in this field can be found in *The British Society of Periodontology - the first 25 years*, commencing therein on page 45. I was one of the founder members of this society. During my time on the staff, we presented various demonstrations at BDA annual conferences and I published a number of papers.

Shortly after my return to London, I was, as already mentioned, appointed as Senior Dental Registrar at St George's Hospital, Hyde

Park Corner, my time then being divided between this appointment and my teaching post at the Royal. When a Senior Dental Hospital Officer post became available at Highlands Hospital, Winchmore Hill, only three miles from home, I decided to apply. I was successful with my application and shortly afterwards took up my new post there. Full details of the developments of the dental department at this hospital are to be found in appendix 11 - *Development of the Dental Department of a General Hospital since the Introduction of the NHS* (British Dental Journal 107323, Dec 1, 1959). I was secretary of the medical committee of the hospital for several years and served as president of the North West London Hospital Group of the BDA in 1960 shortly before we moved to the Midlands.

Following the extension of the Piccadilly Underground line in the late '30s, many new houses were built in and around Southgate, one of the areas under development being Cockfosters. When we moved there it was still a quiet north London village with a church, a post office, a pub, a few shops, and a cricket green with a very active cricket club but, with much post-war development, it was now gradually becoming a thriving suburb of London, with many of the people living there commuting daily to either the City or the West End.

The founder of the church, Christ Church, was Robert Bevan. He came from a Quaker family, was educated at Harrow and Trinity College, Oxford, and became a partner in a great banking house in the City of London. He was in business there for sixty years. By building Christ Church, Cockfosters (which was consecrated in April 1839), Robert Bevan saved the residents of the newly formed Parish of Trent, the long walk to their parish church at Enfield. His heart was turned to God when he was quite young and he was very aware, right from the early days of his conversion, of his responsibility as one of the Lord's stewards. This led to him being a generous supporter not only of his own church, but also of many missions both at home and overseas. He died in 1890 but it was apparent when we joined the congregation that his example had not been forgotten.

The inside of the original building was very different to that which we knew. The east boundary of the church was Chalk Lane and here there was a semi-circular chancel. At the west end of the church there had been a gallery for the organ, choir and Sunday scholars and, as still existed at Holy Trinity, Eastbourne, gated pews. A major enlargement, transforming the interior, was undertaken in 1898. At this time, an aisle was added, along with a transept on the north side; the pews were turned around to face west, the gallery was removed and a new chancel, choir stalls and an organ loft were created at this west end. The other addition was a new vestry. The whole procedure resulted in the seating capacity being increased to 465.

The vicar of this very fashionable North London church was Prebendary Bertram Cecil Hobson, who had been the incumbent since 1921. The church was well known for its floral arrangements and its musical tradition, and many attended from a wide area because of this. At one time, the large, robed choir included four professional salaried members, but only two remained after the war, a bass and a tenor. The vicar's wife, a strict disciplinarian, ensured that not only did choir members attend regularly, but their attire, particularly their shoes and ladies stockings, were black. The display of ladies' hats on Easter Sunday morning, however, simulated something out of *Vogue*!

Although the vicar had served as a chaplain to the forces in the First World War, he became an ardent pacifist and I was told that this caused considerable disquiet when he preached at parade services when troops were billeted in Trent Park during World War II. A feature of his services was the quiet period for reflection after the reading of the lessons.

In 1933, a very large church house had been built adjacent to the church, which was an obvious asset to parish life. This was a large brick building with a main hall suitable for badminton and other games, a stage equipped with theatre stage lighting, two smaller halls, a well equipped kitchen, and other amenities. Not only was it used for special church functions, but it could also be hired by other local organisations. The beautiful words, 'By love serve one another' were engraved above the main entrance.

Soon after we arrived in Cockfosters, a grand, week-long missionary exhibition, supported by various local churches, was organised in this building. I was given the responsibility of arranging all the stewarding. This helped me to meet many members of both our own congregation, as well as people from many other Christian communities in the area.

The precept set by the founder of the church was never lost and when we joined the congregation, several of its members were already on the overseas mission field, whilst others were at training college. Every year a missionary weekend was held during the summer months, with a garden party on the vicarage lawn and speakers from various missionary societies. Fund-raising activities over this weekend, along with offerings given at the Sunday services, raised well over £1,000 each year. This we donated to the missionary societies for the furthering of their work, both here in the UK as well as overseas, particularly those societies in which members of the church were engaged.

Soon after we moved to our flat, the vicar called on us to ask if I would become scoutmaster to the flourishing parish scout troop. Although my uncle had been a District Commissioner in Kent, and my late cousin Bill had been a patrol leader in his troop in Leytonstone, I declined, as I had just been elected as co-leader of the New Barnet Crusader class and also, I had little knowledge of scouting. This decision was a blessing in disguise, as the scoutmaster who was eventually appointed was so successful in the role that the troop had to build their own scout hut to provide sufficient accommodation for all their activities. The troop, along with other uniformed organisations, produced a very lively Gang Show each year. This was supported by many people over a very wide area.

Crusaders played a very important role in my life during these years in Cockfosters. I was involved in many local class activities, firstly at New Barnet, then Whetstone (after we combined the two classes), and finally, after our marriage, at Potters Bar. I was also involved in various Crusader Union activities. The early '50s saw the revival of the annual union sports day, held at the University of London Sports Ground at Motspur Park. I was a gate steward each year, eventually being elevated to chief steward. The annual union rallies, held in Central Hall, Westminster, were also revived as soon as wartime restrictions permitted. This was an event when all the classes within easy reach of central London, and some from the

Home Counties and more distant areas, gathered together for a great service of praise and thanksgiving. Here again I acted as a steward and then became chief steward, part of my role being the counting of the freewill offering after the service.

In 1956 we had our 50th anniversary celebration, which took place in the Royal Albert Hall. There was an afternoon and an evening meeting and not only did this involve organising a large number of stewards, but Beryl and I had the task of counting a very large collection, consisting mainly of small value coins from young class members. It was a wonderful event and the hall staff were amazed at the size of the young audience and their good behaviour.

Canon Hobson died just after Christmas 1949 and there followed a very long interregnum. Many activities introduced at this time and over the next few years, became a regular part of church life. In the early weeks of the interregnum, the Rev Douglas Clark, who was the priest-in-charge at the daughter church, St Paul's, Hadley Wood, introduced a mid-week meeting for bible study and prayer, a vital activity that was continued by the next incumbent and his successors.

Eventually, in 1951, the Rev George Duncan moved to join us from his church in Edinburgh. We had a new incumbent. Prior to his ordination in 1938, Rev Duncan had been a travelling secretary for the Scripture Union. He had served his curacy at St James', Carlisle, before being appointed to a large church in Edinburgh that many of the university students attended. His Scottish upbringing resulted in several Scottish traditions being introduced into our church calendar, including a watch night service on New Year's Eve and alternative tunes to some of the hymns, such as Crimond for the 23rd psalm.

It was perhaps not surprising that in the early days of George Duncan's incumbency, a ten-day coach tour to Dunkeld, Perthshire was arranged (costing only £20.00 per person). This was the beginning of many similar holiday trips, as well as day visits to Oxford, Cambridge, and other similar places of interest. An annual church weekend soon became an integral part of the church calendar as well. It was a wonderful opportunity for members of *all* ages to join together in fellowship, bible study, and prayer, in a quiet retreat away from their daily routine. This event was held at various conference centres within a two hour drive of Cockfosters, at such places as Hildenborough Hall, Frinton-on-Sea and the House of Prayer, Eastbourne. The Youth Fellowship grew in numbers and they too had their weekly annual house party, the first one being at the recently opened Capenwray Hall on the outskirts of the Lake District.

In these early post-war years there were very few conference centres catering for Youth Fellowship groups, so Capenwray Hall was much valued. It had been set up by Major Ian Thomas in an attempt to integrate the youth of Germany and youth of the UK within a Christian environment. Major Thomas had served in the army of occupation following the war and had experienced the difficulties facing many Christian communities in Germany. He realised the great need to involve the Christian youth of both countries. Hence this conference centre, where young people of the two countries could enjoy Christian fellowship together. His great friend Tom Rees had also bought a large mansion after the war which became a conference centre. This was Hildenborough Hall in Kent. Tom Rees also organised monthly Saturday evening youth rallies at the Royal Albert Hall and, much to the amazement of the management, filled the building to capacity on many occasions.

Rev Duncan was a trustee of the Keswick Convention, as had been his father before him. Through his influence, it was not long before Christ Church became involved not only in this convention but also with other, similar local activities. The Keswick Convention was an annual event, held in the Lake District, having first started way back in 1880. The mission statement of this week-long bible ministry affirmed that it was 'committed to a deepening of the spiritual life in individuals and church communities through the careful exposition and application of scripture, seeking to encourage the Lordship of Christ in Life, transformation of the indwelling of the Holy Spirit leading to evangelism, discipleship, and in practical demonstration of Christian unity - All one in Christ Jesus.'

Many churches and missionary societies arranged house parties for this week in Keswick and our church was no exception. Our participation resulted in much blessing for many members of the congregation. These events, together with other factors, soon led to church services becoming very overcrowded and eventually, two services had to be held each Sunday evening.

These were times when many wartime restrictions were beginning to be lifted. A few people now owned a television but programmes were only beamed from Alexander Palace for a few hours each day and were, of course, in monochrome in these early days. Many industries were now benefiting from the technology arising from wartime necessities and this was becoming evident from the products that were now coming on the market. The area that had perhaps the most significance to our church life at this time was in the developments of visual aids. Projectors for 35mm film strips and slides soon became available, as did colour film for 35mm cameras. We were thus able to dispense with the heavy, cumbersome 'magic lantern' and invest in this new, modern equipment.

There were also a large number of 16mm sound film projectors available, these having been used extensively by the forces during the war, both for entertainment and instruction, and now surplus to requirement. We were able to obtain one of these surplus machines through the *Arthur Rank Organisation* and *Religious Films*, replacing it with a more modern instrument a few years later. My experience with our film projector on *HMHS Gerusalemme* was soon put to good use and I hired and showed many of the 16mm films available through missionary societies and other such organisations. *Fact and Faith* films were also entering the market at this time.

One day our vicar was approached by the principal of Oak Hill Theological Collage, part of whose grounds were in our parish, enquiring whether it was possible for a member of their staff, who wished to be ordained, to serve his first curacy at Christ Church. It was proposed that this should be on a part-time basis, so enabling him to continue some of his duties at the college. This was agreed by our PCC and the diocese, and so Ronald Herniman was duly appointed as our curate. This led to a life-long association between our two families that has continued to this day. It also led to closer contact between Christ Church and the college, and more particularly between my family and the college, and we were invited to many of their functions. Many are the contacts that we have had over the years with their past students, some of whom have been the incumbents of parishes in which we have worshipped.

One of the notable events in the Christian calendar of this period was the 1954 Haringay Billy Graham Crusade, held in the very large

Haringay arena, North London, which had a seating capacity of 12,000. Members of Cockfosters congregation helped with this in many different capacities - choir, counsellors and stewards, to name just a few. I was a counsellor and also helped with some of the follow-up visits, and my mother was in the choir.

There was a great publicity programme leading up to the event itself and part of this involved the showing of the Billy Graham film *Oil Town USA* in many venues around London. One of these venues was our own church house and we had showings of the film each evening for a whole week, with three showings on the Saturday. We used both our own projector and that of Oak Hill Theological College, with the principal of the college, the Rev L.F.E. Wilkinson, helping as a projectionist on a number of evenings. Towards the end of the week the hall was packed, with not one empty seat.

The crusade itself was something I shall never forget. On entering the arena one could not miss the cubic mobile hanging from the roof with the text 'I am the Way, the Truth, and the Life' printed on each face. The 'theme hymn' for the Crusade became 'Blessed Assurance - Jesus is mine!' and the first four words of the refrain were emphasised by a special musical rendering:

> *THIS IS MY STORY, this is my song*
> *Praising my Saviour all the day long,*
> *This is my story, this is my song,*
> *Praising my Saviour all the day long.*

It was originally envisaged that the crusade would last for four weeks and the arena had been booked for this period, but so large were the attendances, with the arena being filled to capacity on most evenings, that it continued for almost three months. On the final night, the number wishing to attend was so great, and the queue that formed outside several hours before the meeting was due to commence so vast that, in the interests of public safety, the police broadcast messages requesting that all but ticket holders should stay away. To lessen the disappointment of those without tickets, a large open-air gathering was held at the Wembley Stadium the following evening to cope with this response.

Counsellors were specially trained for the event, attending weekly training sessions for a month or so before the beginning of the crusade. Their main role was to accompany each person who had responded to Billy Graham's appeal at the close of the meeting into the counselling room and, after completing a card with the particulars of the responder, make sure that they understood their commitment to Christ, pray with them, and then introduced them to one of the advisors (a senior member of the Christian community).

The whole crusade, from months beforehand to years after its conclusion, was bathed in prayer, and many are the testimonies of the effectualness of this fervent prayer. 'To God be the Glory.'

Our Marriage - The Braden Family

Beryl and I met when we were both members of the Cockfosters Youth Fellowship at Christ Church and were married in that church by the Rev George Duncan on 3rd September 1955. He was assisted on the day by Rev John Blyth, the curate and minister of our daughter church at Hadley Wood. Mr Duncan spoke on the text 'Not two, but one' from Ephesians, chapter 5. The organist was Mr Roy Slack and we had a full choir who sang an anthem during the signing of the register.

This was a naval wedding, and my best man was Lieutenant Commander James Bonney (my cousin's husband). Their young son, Robert, attired in period naval uniform, was our pageboy. Beryl had three bridesmaids. Two were friends from the church, Gwen Owen and Beryl Hales, and the third, Rachael Harvey, was a Clarendon School colleague who, like Beryl, had also trained as a nurse. My great friend and fellow dental surgeon, Raymond Bird, rang the church clarion as we left the church.

There were about 100 guests and after the marriage service, the vicar kindly allowed us to gather on the vicarage lawn where there were the usual photographs and, unbeknown to me, a short 9.5 mm film was shot by an old naval friend, Vic Simons. We then retired to the church house for a formal wedding breakfast.

One of the speeches at the breakfast was given by Beryl's father, who reminded us that Beryl was a precious stone, a jewel of sea-green colour, one of the foundation stones of the New Jerusalem as portrayed in the last chapter of The Revelation of St John the Divine. (This is also mentioned in several books of the Old Testament, including Song of Solomon, Ezekiel and Daniel). In true naval style, we cut the wedding cake with my sword.

We spent the first night of our honeymoon in Southampton and in the morning, attended the Sunday service at Above Bar Church. The minister there, the Rev Leith Samuel, was an old friend of Will Matheson, with whom I had spent much of my spare time when we were fellow officers on *HMS Collingwood*. The Samuel and Matheson families had organised the Port St Mary CSSM summer mission for many years. In the afternoon we went by ferry to Cowes, Isle of Wight, and had a bus ride to Newport, returning to our hotel in Southampton for dinner.

On the Monday, we drove to Cornwall, spending the rest of the fortnight at a hotel in Fowey. On the way home we bought some home necessities at *Beales* in Plymouth before proceeding to Exeter, where we spent the night at the *Trust House Hotel*.

Due to an impossible landlord, we spent a rather unhappy eighteen months in a flat in Palmers Green, eventually having to leave there on the advice of our solicitor, even though the two-year lease agreement had not expired. Fortunately, the father of my brother-in law Douglas Edmonds was able to invite us to spend the final six months of the lease period in his house nearby whilst the building of our new house was completed.

I found this new property when I was driving to one of our outlying hospitals one day, visiting an elderly patient who had broken her dentures. Driving through the outskirts of Potters Bar, I passed an estate where new houses were being built by *John Laing Company*. I made some enquiries and found that there was a detached house on a large corner plot that was still available. After discussing matters with Beryl we both visited the site on the following Saturday and decided to buy it, providing a mortgage could be obtained through brokers recommended to us by the builders. All went well and we moved there in 1957. We had to purchase all new furniture as this was our first real home, so we had a great time at the annual Ideal Home Exhibition. My father helped to develop the garden and, despite the clay soil, we were able to grow both flowers and vegetables and won several prizes in the Highlands Hospital annual flower show.

Like most other people, we did not have a television at this time but, when we could afford it, we hired one. This helped us to keep up-to-date with various soap operas and to hold more intelligent conversations with our younger patients, all of whom seemed to take television as part of their way of life. We also bought our first sheltie (Shetland sheep dog) and have always had at least one sheltie in our family ever since. In 1960, our son Jonathan was born.

There were many young children on the estate and very few went to Sunday school. We discussed the problem with two of our friends who were teachers and we commenced holding a Sunday school in our own home on Sunday afternoons. We called on all the local families with children to invite their offspring to join us, which proved to be very successful and much appreciated.

When we moved to Potters Bar, I transferred my Crusader leadership to the Potters Bar class, one which possessed its own Crusader hall, making the leadership up to four. Soon after Jonathan was born, I started taking him out in his pram on a Sunday afternoon so that he did not disturb the Sunday school, which did not make me very popular with the other leaders.

* * * * *

Beryl's father, William Eric Braden (known as Eric), was managing director of a tea blending company called *Reddings*, a subsidiary of *Williams Brothers*, a chain of grocery and provision stores in north and east London, and in Essex. This was before the days of instant tea in tea bags, and they blended the tea to give the best taste for the various types of water of the many water companies in London and the Home Counties. The tea was provided in packets for selling in *Williams Brothers* stores and various other outlets. It was also used by some of the airlines.

It was in the early days of his association with this firm that he, Eric, met his future wife, Elsie Kimber, a member of the head office staff. They were married in 1926.

During Beryl's childhood, her father was an active member of an independent church in Harringay, north London, becoming an elder and eventually taking full responsibility following the retirement of the elderly pastor. During the latter years of their lives, Eric and Elsie lived with Beryl's sister and her husband in

Hitchin, Bedfordshire. Elsie died on 23rd March1984 following an asthma attacked (an illness from which she had suffered for much of her life), and Eric died a few years later on 30th August 1987.

Beryl's grandfather, Bernard Ashley Braden, was employed by one of the many gas companies around London before they amalgamated to become the *Gas Light and Coke Company*. He rose to become a senior official of this company. When the family moved from Wilesden to Chesham Bois, he became a very active member of the Amersham (on the hill) Free Church, previously a small mission church that belonged to the Congregational Church of England, the Anglican Church of England, and the Baptists, and was probably the Iron Room, seating 100, which was opened in 1889 on The Moor. This may seem at first to be a rather odd mix of denominations but such a union was quite common in this era. The Baptist Union, as we know it today, was founded much later. Each of the churches was originally an independent body of Christian believers who believed in baptism by immersion, and who chose their own pastor. Grandpa's congregation eventually became a participating member of the Fellowship of Independent Evangelical Churches.

In 1915, a new constitution and set of revised church rules were adopted. These included clauses stating that new members had to be interviewed and then approved at a church meeting. Those not attending communion at least once every six months were removed from membership! Following the appointment of a Minister in 1924 these rules were revised allowing the ordinance of Baptism.

In that same year, a church schoolroom was erected, and in 1917 an organist was appointed. He was a Mr Palmer from Westcliffe-on-Sea and had a stipend of £15.00 per annum. No mention of a pastor is found in the church records before 1924, but in that year the Rev Adam Waugh (from Wallasey, Cheshire) was invited to become their pastor with a stipend of £350.00 per annum and £50.00 towards moving expenses. He accepted and commenced his ministry in Amersham on 5th October.

Bernard Braden was a joint secretary of the Committee of Oversight for several years and is reported in the Amersham *Advertise and Gazette*, the May 1st 1931 edition, as being 'chairman of the Amersham Brotherhood and a prominent deacon of the Free Church'. He was also treasurer to this church in 1924.

Early in 1925, it was agreed that consideration should be given to the building of a new church dedicated to the memory of Alfred Ellis, a previous chairman of the Committee of Oversight. A fund, 'The Alfred Ellis Memorial Church Building Fund', was established, with Mr Braden as its first chairman. During the following years this fund grew considerably, so much in fact that in 1961 it amounted to £10,000 (the original aim was to raise £5,000 for a new church, although building costs would likely have increased and absorbed some of the additional amount).

I am sure that Bernard Braden had many other strings to his bow and we know for a fact that one of them was the Paddington Sick and Provident Club. This is documented in an illustrated address, signed by 59 members, which was presented to him on his retirement as their secretary on the 6th June 1947. We also know that he spent happy years in retirement in Putney, West London, and died in 1956.

Beryl's great great grandfather, the Rev William Braden, was a Congregational minister. He married Agnes Dukes, the eldest daughter of Joshua Dukes. Agnes' brother, Edwin Joshua Dukes, was also a Congregational minister and served as a missionary in China with the London Missionary Society. On his return to the UK, he led several congregations, including a church at Weston-super-mare, and later, Christ Church, Friern Barnet, where an oil painting of him hangs in the vestry.

William Braden was a well known and much sought after preacher and, following his death at the early age of 37, his wife published a book of his sermons. He preached his first sermon at the Bunyan Meeting, Bedford, when he was just 18. His theological studies were carried out at Chesunt College (principal, Dr. Reynolds) and his first pastorate was at St Albans, Hertfordshire. This was followed by a post at Hillhouse Chapel, Huddersfield, during the period 1866-1871, and he finally served at King's Wargh House Chapel in the City of London, located in the same street as my father's offices.

As well as his leadership and preaching, he was very active in the school, the young men's societies, the choral society, and other branches of church work. Unfortunately his health was failing and, on the advice of his physician, he went to America for two months to occupy the pulpit of Dr Soudder in Brooklyn, it being thought that the sea trip would be beneficial to his health. On his return he continued with his duties at the chapel and also with his editorial role on the *English Independent*, but sadly he succumbed to the physical suffering of many years and died from a heart attack the following year.

There were other ordained ministers of the church in the Dukes family. Several members entered the medical profession, with at least two of them having very interesting careers. One of these was Dr Clement Dukes, a well known member of the profession with a worldwide reputation on the health of schoolboys. He qualified from St Thomas' Hospital in 1869 and was appointed as doctor to Rugby School two years later, a post in which he served for 37 years. He wrote several books and in his last work in 1901, entitled *The Fourth Disease*, he attempted to establish the existence of a febrile syndrome which was accompanied by a rash similar to that of measles, rubella, or scarlet fever but, he believed, distinct from them. This became known as 'Dukes Disease'. Although most paediatricians considered it to be a variant of measles or scarlet fever, the entry 'Dukes Disease' appeared in medical dictionaries for many years.

Dr C.E. Dukes OBE FRCS (Eng.), the son of the Rev Edwin Joshua Dukes, was also a member of the profession and a memorial service for himself and his wife, also a doctor, was held at All Souls, Langham Place, London W1 in March 1977.

We know very little of Beryl's maternal grandfather, Harry Kimber. He was born in 1864 and was serving in the Royal Navy in 1891 when he is recorded as having married Sarah Jane Horsley. Members of his family state that he was a deep sea diver and early in his married life suffered from 'the bends'. Although he survived this accident, he suffered from classical ongoing effects of the trauma - chest infections, circulatory problem, and brain damage. It would appear that he was never able to follow any steady employment and he died in a mental institution in 1907.

There were six children from the marriage - Henry Archibald (who died from wounds in World War I), Gertrude Clara, Elsie Eva (Beryl's mother), Marie Emma, William, and Harry Edward. Due to her husband's lack of steady employment, Sarah found it a struggle to keep the family together and they suffered in many ways.

I have not attempted to give a full history of the Braden family as I know that others are researching this. A more detailed account of the Dukes' family history can be found in *Family Dukes - Yesterday* by Cuthbert E. Dukes. One fact that is of historical interest is that the father of a family member called Esquire Dukes was a Thames waterman at the end of the 18th century.

There are also other details which are of importance to present members of the Braden family. In 1918, for example, Ashley Dukes, who was a playwright and brother of Dr C.E. Dukes, married Marie Rambert, the well known ballet dancer who became a DBE in 1962. In her obituary in *The Times* in 1982, Fernau Hall describes her as 'reviver of English ballet'. Another brother, Paul Henry, renowned lecturer and writer, was a spy in Russia during the early days of the Soviet Republic from 1918-1920. He was knighted in 1922.

Many of the Dukes were also schoolteachers, including Joshua, who had his own school in Hackney, East London. In 1841 he married Mary Anne Ashley who was the daughter of Samuel Ashley, a solicitor practising in Tokenhouse Yard, City of London, and a relative of the Shaftsbury family. It would appear that this is where the name Ashley was introduced into the family.

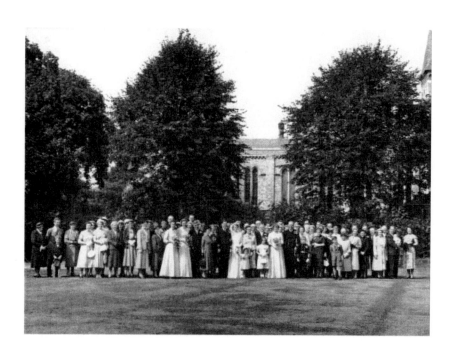

Our wedding at Christchurch, Cockfosters, 3rd September 1955

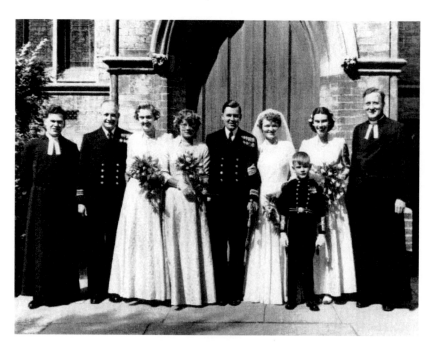

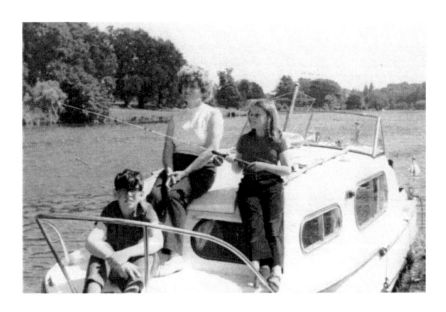

Beryl, Jonathan and Elizabeth on Mia Roma

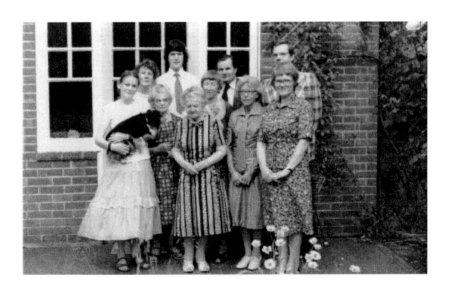

Mother's 90th birthday party at Leigh Cottage, Witley,
2nd July 1979
Front row: Elizabeth (with dog), Auntie Stella, Mother, Mary,
Connie, Beryl
Back row: Joan, Jonathan, John, Robert

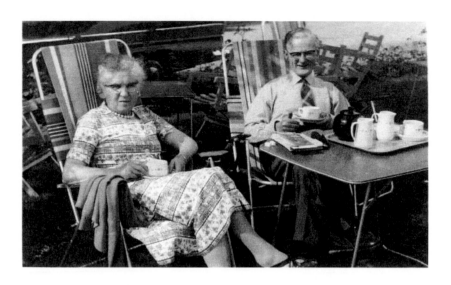

Beryl's parents Eric and Elsie Braden

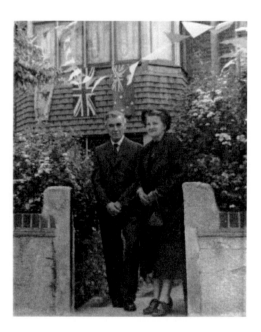

Father and mother outside our house in
Cockfoster's which was decorated for
the coronation of Elizabeth II, 1953)

Back To Our Roots

In 1961, I was successful in gaining an appointment as Senior Hospital Dental Officer (Orthodontics) with the Birmingham Regional Hospital Board. We had done much soul searching before deciding to make this application for, as well as leaving both our families in north London, we had the problem of selling our house and moving to an area where property was very scarce. We also had a very young child, Jonathan being only 18 months old at the time.

After my interview, I made some enquires of estate agents in both Bromsgrove and Worcester, but with little result. I was about to drive home to Potters Bar when I saw, by chance, an advertisement about a property on a new estate in Bromsgrove. I drove over there at once. The estate was in Old Station Road, opposite the playing fields of Bromsgrove School and backing on to the local recreation ground. It was late afternoon and the builders were about to finish work for the day but were able to show me a new detached property from which the prospective buyers had withdrawn that same day. I immediately telephoned the company's head office in Birmingham and reserved the site. I also telephoned Beryl with the news (no mobile phones in those days!) Building was at the stage where we could make certain modifications to suit our needs, and we decided to extend the central heating system. By the time all the legal formalities had been completed, the house was ready for us to move in.

So I joined my new dental team, making the number up to four; two consultants and two senior hospital dental officers. We provided orthodontic advice and treatment within a region that stretched from Shrewsbury in the north to Hereford in the south; a vast area to cover bearing in mind that the construction of motorways around Birmingham had only just begun. At first, I visited weekly clinics at hospitals in Birmingham (Selly Oak), Bromsgrove, Hereford, Kidderminster, and Worcester, with West Bromwich and Stourbridge being added later. When I covered colleagues on leave, I sometimes travelled as far as Shrewsbury. We worked as one harmonious team and one important development at this time was the formation of the Midland Orthodontic Society, the first such regional society in the country; I was one of their early presidents and a presidential badge was presented during my term of office.

One of our consultants, Arnold Huddurt, was undertaking research on the early treatment of cleft palate in babies. This was a fascinating and important study that involved visits to the regional plastic centre and, on one Saturday morning a month, we all met for a cleft palate clinic at Dudley Road Hospital, Birmingham. This research resulted in much advancement in the treatment of this hereditary condition.

There was much to be done in both the house and garden, where we constructed a small pond and a sandpit for Jonathan; we also purchased from a Birmingham store a set of garden swings, rope ladder, etc. We hired a new washing machine which went wrong and boiled all the baby clothes ruining many of them, but fortunately the machine's manufacturer replaced most of them. Having arranged with the builder to supply a larger boiler than was included in the original specifications, we were eventually able to extend the central heating to the bedrooms. One exciting project was the building of a '00 gauge' model railway around Jonathan's bedroom. This was naturally of great interest to father as well as son, and kept them both well occupied! Many years before this, the railways of Britain had been nationalised and the liveries of the old companies had disappeared. Diesel traction was replacing steam and colour light signalling was being introduced on many sections. These changes were reflected in our layout.

The railway line from Bromsgrove to Birmingham had a steep incline, called the Lickey Incline, and many steam trains proceeding north from Bromsgrove required a backing engine to help them on their way. This was of great interest to Jonathan as he watched from his pushchair on our frequent visits to the station.

In 1963, Elizabeth was born. Beryl was thus kept very busy at home. Our next door neighbours also had a young baby and so we were able to share baby-sitting. It was also around this time that Beryl took driving lessons. Previous to this, she had held a motorcycle licence for many years. The lessons were a success and Beryl passed her test.

Whilst living in Potters Bar, before Jonathan was born, Beryl and I had spent a caravan holiday in South Devon and, with our now growing family, we decided that we should take up caravanning for our holidays. After visiting numerous caravan dealers in the area we eventually bought our first small, rather ancient caravan for £70.00. Our friends, Ron and Grace Herniman, who were experienced in towing caravans, very kindly offered to tow it to a site we had reserved near Towyn in North Wales. As this was only a two hour drive from home, it meant that we could get away for long weekends as well as summer holidays.

It was not long before we purchased a larger van on the same site, from which we could see the trains on the Tallylyn railway. Later we exchanged our static van for a touring van and this enabled us to drive all over the country, ranging from Dornoch and Aviemore in Scotland, to various places in Devon and Cornwall. We also attended a number of Caravan Club rallies.

During this period, we developed a routine whereby we usually went up to London for Christmas, enabling us to visit both our families. My mother and father then came to stay with us at Easter and Beryl's parents visited us at other times of the year.

I continued to attend the monthly meetings in London of the BSSO, usually travelling by car on the newly opened M1 motorway, stopping for an early evening meal with my parents in Cockfosters before continuing to central London. The return journey in the late evening only took just over two hours, as the motorway was nearly empty once you had passed the Dunstable junction. In the winter, when the weather was poor, I usually travelled by train from Birmingham Snow Hill to Paddington on a new multiple diesel train, the first to be introduced to Britain, returning on a later train from Euston to Birmingham New Street, with a change at Rugby. I was able to garage the car near Snow Hill station for the afternoon.

As a family, we attended the local Methodist church for their morning service, as it was a long uphill walk with prams to the parish church where I usually attended evensong. It was a very small evening congregation compared with Cockfosters. I was elected to the PCC and we became friends with the recently appointed curate and his wife. They had just had their first baby and we were able to share with them our experiences as new parents.

Soon after we moved to Bromsgrove, the general secretary of *Fact & Faith Films*, knowing that I had had experience with film projection in both the navy and in Cockfosters, invited me to be their West Midlands Regional Secretary. I was provided with the necessary projection equipment and was soon travelling around the area, on average about one evening a week, presenting their scientific films, which had been produced by the Moody Bible Institute of America. It was very interesting deputation work.

Just after commencing this work, I was asked by Jack Watford, the secretary of the Crusader Union, if I would help with the leadership of the Kidderminster class. I declined as I was already travelling many miles each week by car and I felt that this extra 30-mile round trip would be too much for me and would also take away time that I wanted to spend with the family.

Word of my experience as a projectionist got around and I was asked by the very active Arts group in Bromsgrove if I would project some of the special films they had hired for their summer festival on our projector. The *Fact & Films* central committee agreed to this, providing I could also project some of their films at the event. This joint co-operation thus resulted in an interesting outreach opportunity.

With a growing family we decided that, to supplement our income, we would respond to Birmingham University's request for accommodation for students and so two such students occupied our spare room for two years on a B&B basis.

* * * * *

Around this time, The Open University was developing and Beryl and I became two of their early students, she commencing with a foundation course in humanities, whilst I chose a similar course with the Science Faculty. With so many changes and advances having been made in the sciences since I left school, including new teaching methods and many new discoveries, this proved invaluable to me when Jonathan and Elizabeth started studying these subjects at school.

We both received our degree at a graduation ceremony in the Central Hall, Westminster, London, in 1975, when we were living in Surrey. This proved to be quite an eventful day as just before the ceremony, we received a telephone call from Jonathan's school to report that he had been taken to hospital after diving into the swimming pool and hitting his head on the bottom! Fortunately all was well so we travelled home via Leatherhead so that we could take him home with us.

Since moving to the Midlands, we had always felt that we would like to live in Malvern in Worcestershire. Beryl had spent two years there during the latter part of the war and had fallen in love with the countryside around the hills. Now that my clinics were more concentrated around this area, and we discovered that there was more choice of schools for Jonathan and Elizabeth who were both fast approaching school age, we decided to look for a property in that area. Eventually we found a suitable house in St Andrews Road, close to the Royal Radar Establishment. This proved to be a very wise decision as, not only were our children happy at school there, but we were blessed with the worship at Malvern Priory Church. The area also had a wide variety of amenities which we were able to enjoy as a family.

This house was much larger than our Bromsgrove one and in a very convenient position. Jonathan and Elizabeth soon made friends with the next-door children who were about the same age. When they all reached school age we were able to car share with their parents for school journeys. There was much decoration required in the house and reconstruction of the garden which had been rather neglected over the years. We brought all the garden climbing frames, etc. with us and these were much appreciated by Jonathan's new friends. We terraced the garden, which already had some fruit trees in it, and constructed a new pond. In place of an old broken-down wooden stable, we installed a new garage with room for both cars. There was plenty of room at the side of the house for our caravan.

The move also gave me wider opportunities in my work with *Fact & Faith Films* and eventually led to Christian outreach at the Three Counties Agricultural Show, which was held each year at their permanent site on the outskirts of the town. We had a tent at the show where we projected various films to the crowds in attendance. Our first activity was on the Sunday afternoon whilst exhibitors were erecting their stands prior to the official opening, when the show committee permitted us to hold an open air service in the bandstand.

This event started a trend for similar outreach with the films by other members of the society at similar agricultural shows and a tent at the Royal Agricultural Show at Stoneleigh soon became an annual fixture. When we moved to Surrey I was able, with the help of Christian leaders in the neighbourhood, to establish a tent at the Guildford Agricultural Show.

During the summer months, a local group of church leaders invited the many visitors in the town, by means of posters in hotels and shops and notices at church services, to showings of these films at the local council offices. These were well attended and much appreciated by visitors and residents alike.

Beryl and I soon became involved in the activities of Malvern Priory Church; Elizabeth attended the morning service with us whilst Jonathan joined in with their Pathfinder class which was held in the nearby upper room of the church hall at the same time. As soon as he was old enough, Jonathan also attended the Malvern Crusader class on Sunday afternoons, and went to his first Crusader house party at their centre, *Westbrook*, in Ryde, on the Isle of Wight. This centre had been established in memory of those past Crusaders who had died during the Second World War. When she was old enough, Elizabeth joined the girls' class.

It was not long before I was elected to the PCC and offered the role of sidesman, occasionally being asked to read one of the lessons. I was also appointed to the Deanery Synod some time later and was one of their representatives on the Diocesan Board of Finance and their Diocesan Retreat House committee.

We had been caravanning for many years but, as we were now living near Tewekesbury where the River Avon flowed into the River Severn, we sold our caravan and purchased a small *Freeman* motor cruiser, *Mia Roma*, berthing her at a new marina on the Avon near Tewkesbury. She gave us all many hours of pleasure, and both Jonathan and Elizabeth became very efficient as crew members. We made this purchase knowing that we would probably have to sell her to pay for school fees and this eventually proved to be the case, prompted by rocketing inflation in the 1970s.

There was a good train service from Malvern to London and I was able to travel there to attend the monthly meetings of the BSSO and also, with the M5 motorway having now been extended north of Birmingham, it was an easy journey by car to the monthly meeting of the Midland Orthodontic Society.

It was during our time in Malvern that my mother heard that Auntie Agnes, one of her sisters, had been admitted to hospital in Eastbourne with a serious condition. We knew that she had had an operation at the Middlesex Hospital for cancer of the bowel many years earlier, and she had often been in considerable pain when she visited us in Cockfosters. It was becoming increasingly difficult for my parents to travel long distances, so it was fortunate that I was able to combine attendance at my next BSSO meeting with a visit to Auntie Agnes in hospital. I was able to discuss her situation with the ward sister and I learnt that her condition was terminal. She died a few days later.

* * * * *

Unfortunately, changes were brewing at work which were to have consequences for both myself and the family. It was decided by the Regional Hospital Board that the overall workload carried by our team necessitated the appointment of a third orthodontic consultant who, on appointment, took over from the consultant in my part of the region with whom I had shared clinics for almost ten years. The new consultant's approach to orthodontics in general, and to me in particular, was such that it made my work untenable, and also caused much concern to the local general dental practitioners who very much appreciated both the services we had provided in the past and our orthodox seminars. We were no longer working as one harmonious team and I had no option but to seek employment elsewhere.

Fortunately, I secured an appointment as an orthodontist to the Surrey County Council, based in Guildford, although it was at a much reduced salary. Once again we had the problem of finding a suitable house as there was still a housing shortage in the area. We eventually purchased one in Godalming. We moved just before Christmas 1971 and then, together with my mother and father, stayed at Lee Abbey, Lynton, for their Christmas house party. In January, Jonathan returned to his school near Malvern to spend two terms as a boarder as he was within a few months of sitting his common entrance exam.

The family were very sorry to leave the Midlands as we had been very settled in the area and Beryl and I, as well Jonathan and Elizabeth, had made many friends. There was also the fact that my mother and father had moved to Malvern to be near us.

Godalmimg, about five miles from Guildford, is a very old Saxon town with a narrow high street. It was one of the staging points on the London to Portsmouth stagecoach route and it was here that they changed the horses before the steep ascent to Hindhead. In 1575, the town was granted its Borough Charter by Queen Elizabeth I.

Much of the development of the town over the centuries has been influenced by the geography of the area. Godalming lies in the valley of the River Wey, a tributary of the River Thames, where the course of the river cuts through an extensive outcrop of bargate stone, a local division of the Hythe beds. The old town grew between the flood plain and the surrounding hills.

Due to the fact that much of the land was too poor for cultivation, the fields around the town were used as pasture land for grazing sheep. Consequently, a woollen industry developed and alongside this, subsidiary industries such as leather dressing and the manufacturing of gloves. All of these activities brought wealth to the town aided by the fact that, with the River Wey being navigable to the outskirts of the town, they had an important transport route to London and beyond. Trade routes were developed even further when the railway from London was extended to the town in 1849 and the Waterloo to Portsmouth line was opened in 1859.

From the 12th century onwards, the quarrying of bargate stone around the town became another important industry and it was still being quarried at the bottom of Shacksted Lane until the outbreak of the Second World War. This stone was used in the construction of many buildings in the town, including the old parish church and the chapel of Charterhouse School.

Although there was still a shortage of housing in the area, and that which was available was much dearer than property in Malvern, we were fortunate enough to obtain a detached house at the top of Shacksted Lane which had coal-fuelled central heating and a garage. Other than converting the central heating to gas and insulating the outside walls, few improvements were necessary. There was a good sized boarded loft complete with loft ladder and there was plenty of room to enable us to reassemble the model railway we had constructed in Bromsgrove. Over the years, we redecorated all the rooms ourselves and employed decorators for the outside painting.

We were able to find a mooring on the Thames for our motor cruiser at Bray, near Maidenhead, just over half an hour drive from Godalming. Later we moved her to Wargrave, a short distance from Henley-on-Thames, fairly near to the Royal Masonic home at Windlesham where my mother was then living. This opened up a much wider choice of waterways for us and we were able to cruise from Letchworth, close to the source of the Thames, and downstream to Staines and beyond. Eventually we decided to move our mooring closer to home on the River Wey near Wisley, Surrey, before having to make the decision to sell the craft.

Elizabeth soon settled at her new school in Godalming and then later, into the Royal Naval School, Haslemere. It was not so simple for Jonathan. When we knew that we were moving to Surrey, we changed his registration from Malvern College to Charterhouse School and we expected all to be well. However, a few weeks before he was due to start at this school, we received a letter from the bursar saying that there had been a muddle with the registration. Regretfully, he informed us, Jonathan's entry date was oversubscribed and they could not accept him. Beryl quickly made frantic telephone calls to other schools in the area and eventually found a place for him at St John's School, Leatherhead, which was close enough to allow him to travel daily by train with only two changes - in those days trains were reliable and various routes interlocked with one another. As time went by, this proved to be a fortuitous move and a better choice for him both academically and socially.

179

Both Jonathan and Elizabeth became involved in Crusader classes in the town and were soon enjoying camps and other summer holiday activities. Jonathan continued the Munns' family sea-going tradition and went on yachting holidays with Crusaders, sailing across the channel to mainland Europe. We all attended the nearby church at Busbridge (rector, the Rev Jack Cresswell), and I was elected to the PCC at the next AGM. Rev Cresswell retired in 1978 and, during the interregnum that followed, I helped with the reading of the lessons, congregational prayers and at communion services. During my time at the church, a church room was built in the old graveyard, the planning of which involved much searching to locate the living relatives of people interned in the graveyard in order to obtain their permission to build on the graveyard.

During the Easter holiday, we went on our first trip abroad as a family, travelling to Europe to visit the Dutch bulb fields. Holiday air travel was in its infancy and we travelled by sea from Dover to Ostend where we stayed for three nights. During our stay, we travelled by coach to see the bulb fields in Holland and the Belgium city of Brugge.

Evensong

With the children growing up, we now needed more space at home, and also a spare bedroom for visits from our parents and families, so we decided to move to a larger house in the Petworth Road, Milford, on the outskirts of Godalming. It had four bedrooms, a large kitchen/breakfast room and a very large loft. Outside there was a garage, parking for a second car, and a moderate sized garden with a greenhouse.

Jonathan, as well as gaining his Duke of Edinburgh award, soon completed his 'O' and 'A' levels, with sufficiently good grades to secure him a place at Guy's Hospital Dental School, University of London, where he soon made friends with various students in Guy's CU. He found digs in a vicarage in Dockland (before all the new developments had commenced) and cycled each day from there to the dental school at London Bridge. We were able to purchase a desk and other furniture from our local house clearance sales and one Saturday, we hired a self-drive van to take these to London. During his time at Guy's, Jonathan also lived in a shared flat in Tulse Hill and a house owned by the father of one of his flatmates in one of London's residential squares near Elephant and Castle.

Elizabeth did well at the Royal Naval School and Godalming Sixth Form College, and secured a university place in York on a science degree course. Initially, she lived in one of the halls of residence but after her first year, she too moved to a house which she shared with some fellow students.

There were some sad times whilst we were in Godalming. Beryl's mother, who had suffered from asthma all her life, had a severe attack and died before the doctor could get to her, he having been delayed in attending her. Her husband, with the help of a son-in-law with whom he was living, was able to make all the necessary funeral arrangements. Then, early one morning, we had a telephone call from my mother to tell us that my father had died during the night from a heart attack. I travelled to Malvern to make all the arrangements for his funeral which was held at the Worcester crematorium a week later.

A few months after my father died, the police called on us one Sunday lunch time to report that my mother's sister, Cissie, had been found dead in her bungalow at Bexleyheath. They had traced us through letters found in her house. It transpired that neighbours, worried that her milk had not been retrieved from her doorstep, had called the police. When the police broke into the house, they found her dead in her chair, having passed away from natural causes.

I, being the only male relative, had to drive to Kent the following day and make all the necessary arrangements. My mother was the senior surviving relative and, as no executors had been appointed, I also organised the sale of the bungalow for her and attended to all the legal formalities. Auntie Cissie died intestate as the only will found was unsigned. This resulted in the assets from the estate being divided amongst her remaining elderly sisters. Many of them were receiving state benefits which were reduced when they received their inheritance, so they were unable to enjoy their windfall to the full. This whole situation demonstrated how important it is to leave a valid will.

Now that the children were no longer in permanent residence at home, we did not need such a large house and we moved to a smaller property in nearby Witley. I became a member of Witley Parish Church and was elected to their PCC, later being nominated as one of their Deanery Synod representatives, and eventually put forward by that body as one of their members on the Guildford Diocesan Synod. I was elected and, whilst carrying out my role, renewed my friendship with my Crusader friend and fellow dental surgeon, John Ruff, who was one of the Dorking Deanery Synod's representatives.

I served on the Synod Schools Committee, eventually becoming one of the governors at Bishop Reindorf Secondary School, one of the two church secondary schools in the diocese. Strangely enough, the mother of the headmaster of this school had been a friend of my mother when they both lived in Cockfosters. I also represented the diocese on panels that were set up to hear appeals from parents who had been denied a place for their child at a primary school of their choice.

The vicar of our new church in Witley was the Rev Philip Case, who was also the rural dean of Godalming. In 1984, he retired to Devon and once again we were involved in a long interregnum during which I officiated at the Sunday evening services. I also liaised with the minister of a nearby parish to arrange weddings and funerals as both the church wardens, who would normally fulfil this role, were out of the area during the daytime. Other activities for which I accepted responsibility were the distribution of the monthly parish magazine and the organising of covenants for the weekly/monthly planned giving. I was also one of the parish representatives on the village hall committee.

Both Beryl and I progressed with our Open University studies and when Beryl had completed her basic degree, she successfully applied to the Sociology Faculty of the University of Surrey to study for a master's degree in social research. This led to her being offered a research appointment at St Joseph's Hospice, East London. The one downside of this was that she then had a four hour train and bus journey each day. On completing her master's degree, she continued her studies with a thesis on 'Quality of Life' for patients who were dying in hospitals and hospices, eventually receiving her doctorate in a ceremony at Guildford Cathedral. By this time, we had moved down to Devon.

There were many changes within the NHS after I was appointed as an orthodontist to the Surrey County Council. Within a year or two of our move, I was transferred to the newly established Surrey Area Health Authority whose headquarters were in Guildford. A Dental Area Committee was convened, with me as their secretary.

For those of us employed in the school dental service, The BDA became the trades union. I was elected as one of their shop stewards for the Surrey area, for which I had to know about certain legal procedures. These I learnt about at a training course at Keele University. I also had to attend various meetings in London. It certainly gave me another interest apart from orthodontics, as well as a deeper insight into the workings of the profession. Also at this time, I was elected to the committee of the BSSO as a representative of orthodontists working within the school dental service.

* * * * *

I finally retired, on reaching the age of 65, in 1984. Beryl, although she was still continuing her studies with the University of Surrey, retired three years later. When I retired, we went on a very interesting river cruise on the River Rhine, travelling through Holland, Germany, France and into Switzerland, where we anchored for two nights in Basle. From there we took a coach trip to Interlaken and beyond.

During these years in Witley, we often visited Beryl's aunt and uncle in Worthing. I also visited my mother's sisters, Auntie Ethel, in Eastbourne, and Auntie Stella, in Hove. On reaching the age of 65, Auntie Ethel had negotiated a rather nice apartment in the Queen Alexander's Homes in Seaside, Eastbourne, and she lived there very happily for many years, continuing to attend the local Girl's Friendly Society meetings as well as being a regular attendee of Holy Trinity Church.

It gradually became obvious to me, on my regular visits to see her, that Auntie Ethel was becoming very frail and, following a short stay in hospital, we had to find a nursing home for her. With the help of the local health visitor, whom I had apparently treated when I was in practice in the town, she was admitted to a very comfortable nursing home. Later, she unfortunately became too incapacitated for them to nurse her and had to be transferred to another home where she died within a few weeks. I took my mother, who was then living at Lord Harris Court, to her funeral at Holy Trinity Church, Eastbourne, which was attended by many of Auntie Ethel's friends. We were most grateful to the vicar and his wife, whom we had known for many years, for their cooperation and hospitality. Auntie Ethel had left a very detailed will, with me as one of the executors, and all the arrangements went smoothly.

One Friday evening Heather, Auntie Stella's daughter, telephoned us to enquire as to whether we had heard from her mother as she could not obtain any reply on the telephone. We hadn't, but as we had planned to visit Beryl's relations the following day we said we would make some enquiries. I left Beryl in Worthing and Jonathan and I drove to Auntie Stella's flat in Hove. We could get no reply at the door so asked the landlord to let us in with his pass key. She was not there which was a bit of a mystery as there was an untouched meal on the table. We then made enquiries at the police station. They knew nothing except that an unidentified lady had collapsed in the street the previous day and been taken by ambulance to hospital. On enquiring at the hospital, we were told that they did have an unidentified patient - she had refused to tell them her name or next-of-kin. This indeed turned out to be Auntie Stella. Mystery solved, but it does emphasize the problems, and the consequent worry and expense, which can be caused when one is so secretive.

On being admitted to the hospital, Auntie Stella had undergone an operation for a fractured hip, having sustained the injury after apparently falling in the street. This left her very disabled and she never recovered sufficiently to enable her to return to her second floor flat, approached as it was by a steep and narrow staircase. She died several months later in another hospital. As her eldest daughter, Ruth, was very disabled herself and lived in Canada, Heather, the youngest daughter, made all the funeral arrangements. Sadly we were also to lose Beryl's uncle, then her father, and finally her aunt whilst we were in Witley. We attended all their funerals.

* * * * *

Jonathan qualified as a dental surgeon in 1983 and we proudly attended his degree ceremony in the Royal Albert Hall. His second house surgeon appointment was at Surrey County Hospital, Guildford, where he met his wife Sue. They were married by the Venerable Ronald Herniman, our old family friend who was also Jonathan's godfather, in Witley Parish Church during the above mentioned interregnum. Two years later, he joined a dental practice in Barnstaple, Devon, and bought a house on the outskirts of the town, where our first grandchild, Hannah, was born. Sadly his marriage broke up and he has now left Barnstaple and is practising in Cornwall.

Our eldest grandchild, Hannah, did very well at school and embarked on a law course at the University of the West of England, Bristol. She has just received her degree (June 2008), and is continuing with her studies at the same university.

Daniel, Hannah's brother, also had a good school result and is just completing his first year on an engineering course at Oxford Brook University. His great love is go-cart racing and he would eventually like to be on a team participating on the premier racing circuits.

Kathryn, the youngest member of the family and our youngest grandchild, has just completed her first year at sixth form college but has yet to decide on her future career path.

Beryl had delayed her retirement because, owing to the regulations at the time, she was unable to count the years she had worked before taking a break when Jonathan and Elizabeth were young. Hence, she still had to work the required number of years before she could claim an NHS pension. Once she had finally retired and we were free to move, we put our house in Witley on the market, soon receiving an exceptional offer. After much thought and consideration, we moved to the small village of Cruwys Morchard, about six miles from Tiverton, Devon, having bought the delightfully named Sunday School Cottage.

The property had been built by the church in the 1840s for the education of the local children during the week (this was before the days of Board Schools), and for other parishioners on Sundays after they had attended the morning service. From our survey report we knew that there was no damp course and we took steps to remedy this. There were a few alterations we wanted to make to the ground floor, including the creation of a modern kitchen, complete with an electric Aga, and an entrance hall with a cloakroom, and we were fortunate in obtaining the services of a local builder for this. We also converted the central heating system from oil to gas. Certain stonework on the front of the building needed replacing and for this we employed the diocesan masons. It was shortly after this work was completed that the building was Grade II listed.

We used our home for many church and village functions, such as Lenten study groups, PCC meetings, and meetings of the Women's Institute, our large front room being much preferred to the rather bare and draughty village hall.

The cottage had a large garden, which kept me well occupied, although the local farmer was thankfully very good in attending to the hedges. One of my projects was the erection of fruit cages where we cultivated raspberries, blackcurrants, and gooseberries. I had been quite keen on gardening ever since I had a small garden of my own in East Sheen, and we developed gardens at all our other houses. I even exhibited at the annual flower & vegetable show at Highlands Hospital. Our interest in gardens and gardening prompted Beryl and I to join the Royal Horticultural Society and we regularly visited the annual Chelsea Flower Show. We also continued our interest in the county shows and became members of the Devon County Show, which we attended each year.

Soon after we moved to Cruwys Morchard, vandals broke down our main wooden, and rather dilapidated, garage door and stole various tools and food from our freezer. With the help of our insurance policy, we were able to replace the doors with modern lockable ones and so increase the security of the estate. We soon learnt the many ways of the countryside and were warned against one individual who, if you did not keep your logs under lock and key, would steal them one night and then try to sell them back to you the next day!

Another member joined our family at this time, a stray cat, who made herself comfortable in our garage and soon became a pet. We also had two Shelties, who had been with us for many years and, whilst in Malvern, we had given a home to two budgerigars following the death of their owner. Our bird population had since been added to and whilst helping with *Fact and Faith Films* at the Stoneleigh Show, I purchased an outdoor aviary.

The new Tiverton Parkway station could be easily reached from our home in about 20 minutes and had a good car park. There was a train service to Reading and Paddington and, with a reliable half-hourly connecting service onwards Reading to Wokingham, I enjoyed comfortable fortnightly journeys to visit my mother (trains were not crowded, except at holiday times), who was by this time well established in a Masonic nursing home near Wokingham, Berkshire. This latter train was on the Reading to Gatwick line and as this passed through Guildford I could easily travel there to fulfil my school manager commitments. I also travelled by train quite often to attend council meetings of the Christian Dental Fellowship as I was responsible for organising their covenant scheme, and later gift aid donations, and raised considerable finances for them. Another good service was the daily, direct service to Edinburgh which was useful for visiting Elizabeth.

$$* \quad * \quad * \quad * \quad *$$

Living in the depths of the countryside, our eyes were opened to the plight of the ministry of the Church of England in the small and scattered parishes. The parish of Cruwys Morchard, a small parish of about 500 souls, of whom the majority were connected with farming, was one of twelve parishes within the Exe Valley Group Ministry (Diocese of Exeter), but which only had two ordained ministers responsible for all of the twelve churches. This meant that there could only be one service in each church on Sundays, with times having to be varied each Sunday to enable one of the two ordained clergy to be present at communion services. This inevitably led to confusion for the villagers on occasions, and the smooth running of the group very much depended on lay readers. Despite the efforts of our vicar, the Rev Harold Witty, the result was that church services were poorly attended and even then, the congregation was mainly composed of members of the PCC. Funeral services, on the other hand, were often attended by anything up to 200 people.

After we had been living in the parish for several years, I was elected as a church warden and it was during my term of office that we had to raise a considerable sum of money for extensive repairs to the church roof. The roof had suffered from poor and make-shift repairs over a number of decades and this had resulted in considerable damage being caused elsewhere in the building. There was little money available either from the diocese or other church sources, partly due to the great financial losses the church commissioners had suffered in the post-war years, and so we had to appeal to whatsoever charities we thought might help us. I had the task of raising funds and, after searching the appropriate books in the county reference library at Exeter, I wrote fifty or more letters to possible donors before we secured the many thousands of pounds we needed to proceed with the repairs.

On 3rd July 1989 we celebrated my mother's 100th birthday, and much celebrating there was. As it was a Sunday, we attended the regular Sunday morning communion service at Lord Harris Court followed by a buffet luncheon in the large lounge. All the residents and our family and friends were invited to this and Jonathan and I prepared a slide sequence of photographs and other memorabilia depicting my mother's life over the preceding 100 years. The climax of this was the singing of one of their school songs by Camden School, New South Wales, Australia, and a congratulatory speech from the mayor of that town. A friend made a video of the whole proceedings. My mother died in her 105th year.

Soon after we moved to Cruwys Morchard, Beryl was invited to become a trustee of Children's Hospice South West based in Barnstaple. At this time, there was only one other children's hospice in the country and, as this was at Oxford, it meant long journeys for those families living in the South West who needed the support it offered. The dream of the trustees was to build a new hospice in North Devon. It was a huge undertaking for, as well as making the people of this area aware of the need for, and the functions of, a hospice for children (a concept that varied considerably from that of hospices for adults), land had to be obtained, architects plans drawn up, and building permission approved - a great deal of work before the dream could become a reality.

Needless to say, the project was a costly one, with almost three million pounds needing to be raised for the building, the initial salaries of nursing and care staff, and a contingency to ensure that the expenses of at least the first year of operating could be met. The result was that Beryl and I, the other trustees, and many others, attended promotional meeting in Devon, Cornwall, Somerset, and beyond, many of them in evenings and at weekends. The hospice was eventually opened in Barnstaple in 1995.

One of Beryl's many duties was to represent the trustees on interviewing panels of staff. My role was more on the financial side and I helped with many aspects of raising funds, particularly with covenants at first and then gift aid when this was introduced by the Chancellor. Beryl served as a trustee for more than 15 years until she finally retired from the role in 2006.

Some ten years previous to this we had come to live near Barnstaple ourselves. The upkeep of our property in Cruwys Morchard had become progressively more expensive and the garden was proving too large to maintain so in 1996, we moved to a smaller house in Fremington, this being much nearer to the hospice. It was also easier to maintain, with a much reduced annual upkeep.

Whilst both of us were still kept busy with duties at the hospice, I was also involved with various duties in church services at the local parish church and was soon elected to the PCC. Beryl was involved in several outside activities, including the North Devon Choral Society. She also completed a two year non-residential course of theology study at Maryvale College, Birmingham, and took a music diploma with the Open University.

We had some interesting holidays whilst living in Fremington, including a cruise to Madeira and the Canary Islands, a cruise on a container/cargo ship which took us across the North Sea, through the Kiel Canal, up the Baltic to Helsinki and beyond (what a change in navigation aids from my wartime experiences on the hospital ship), and a cruise on the *Saga Rose* to ports on the Mediterranean Sea, including those for Florence and Rome. In 2005 we celebrated our 50th wedding anniversary with a family luncheon at a hotel in Coombe Martin, and we held a similar function at the *Tiverton Hotel* for Beryl's 80th birthday.

With neither of us getting any younger, and following much research and visiting of possible locations, we decided that the time had come for us to move to a retirement development. After many promises from the retirement company as to when the buildings would be completed, we eventually moved into Blagdon Village, Taunton, in June 2007. This estate has a very interesting history, at one time being the residence of the Archdeacon of Taunton, then becoming one of the special needs schools of the Dr Barnado Trust who still have an interest in the freehold.

We are now well settled here and in our spiritual home at St Mary Magdalene Parish Church. This year, 2008, the church is celebrating its 700th anniversary as a parish and the 500th anniversary of the present building. The building and the services remind me very much of Mortlake Parish Church. Pews have been removed from the west end of the church to provide both a coffee area (with light refreshments available on most week days) and a large area for the sale of Christian literature and greeting and devotional cards; this is open after the Sunday morning service, and mornings and afternoons Monday to Friday. Many local residents, as well as visitors to the town, use these facilities, with the result that our outreach is not just on Sundays but throughout the week. Beryl helps with the bookstall but, unfortunately, my lack of mobility restricts my activities.

O God, from whom all holy desires, all good counsels, and all just works do proceed: Give unto thy servants that peace which the world cannot give; that both our hearts may be set to obey thy commandments, and also that by thee we being defended from the fear of our enemies may pass our time in rest and quietness; through the merits of Jesus Christ Our Saviour.

Evening Collect

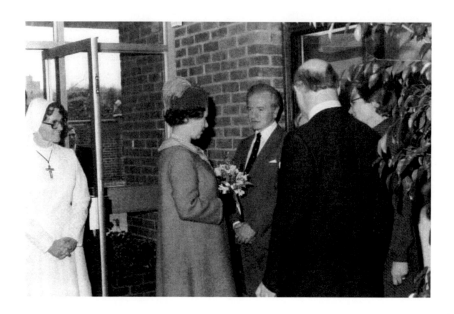

The Queen's visit to St Joseph's Hospice, Hackney, East London.
Beryl *far right*

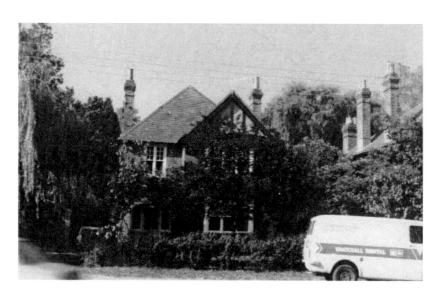

Our home in Petworth Road on the outskirts of Godalming

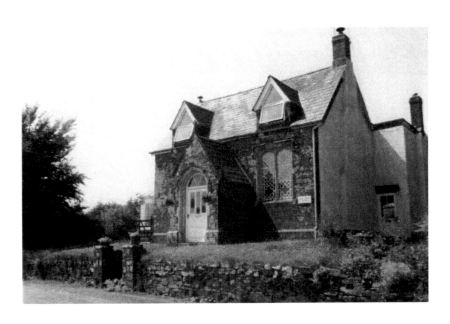

Sunday School Cottage, Cruwys Morchard

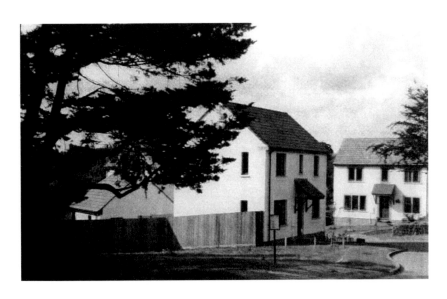

Our house in Beech Park, Fremington

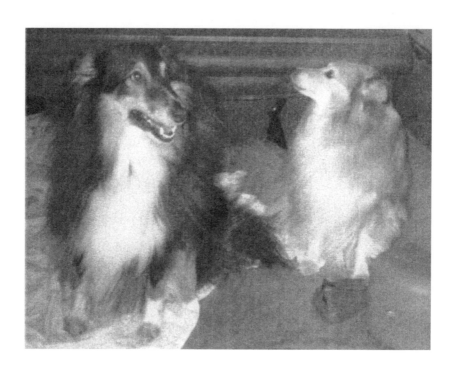

Sheppie and Becky

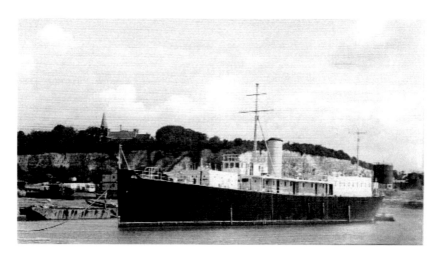

HMS Chrysanthemum

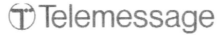

Telemessage

RDG5713 LLX5866 PFC0005 P52 BUCK05   02 JUL 1989/1432

Buckingham Palace
London
SW1A 1AA

02 July 1989

TELEMESSAGE LXP   ROYAL-CARD
MRS. FLORENCE MINNIE MUNNS
LORD HARRIS COURT
MOLE ROAD, SINDLESHAM
WOKINGHAM
BERKSHIRE

I AM DELIGHTED TO SEND YOU MY WARM CONGRATULATIONS ON YOUR
ONE HUNDREDTH BIRTHDAY, TOGETHER WITH MY BEST WISHES FOR AN
ENJOYABLE CELEBRATION.

ELIZABETH R.

Mother's 100th birthday telegram

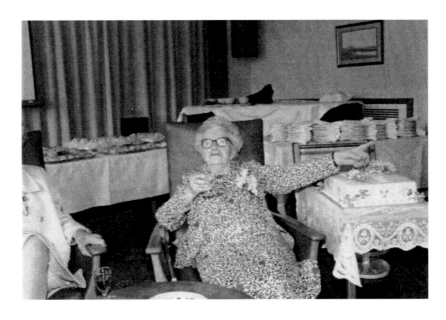

Celebrating mother's 100th birthday

195

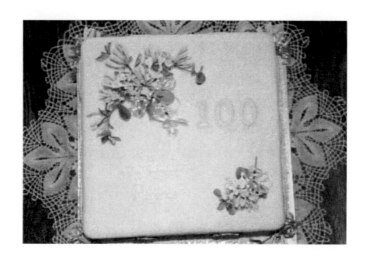

100th birthday cake

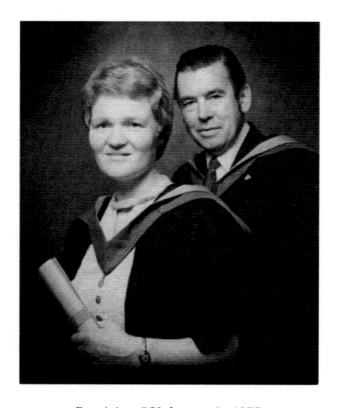

Receiving OU degrees in 1975

Epilogue

The theme of the introduction to this book was change. Have many changes taken place around you during your lifetime? I would be surprised if this has not been the case. The technological development sparked off by the industrial revolution brought immense change to the lives of our grandparents - the coming of the railway and other mechanical means of transportation, the introduction of gas to so many homes where previously there was a coal or wood burning range for cooking and heating and only candles for lighting, the discovery of nitrous oxide and chloroform as anaesthetics. No doubt you could name many more life-changing discoveries and inventions.

In the lifetime of my generation, the greatest development has probably been the harnessing and application of electricity. With so many of our modern facilities dependent on electricity (communications, transport and media presentation, to name just a few), it is hard to imagine how we would manage without it now. We must also remember the many advances in medical research resulting in the discovery of penicillin, and the developments of the many drugs upon which all of us in the developed countries of the world depend today. Are we, each one of us, doing our best to provide these advantages to others throughout the world, particularly those who are less fortunate than ourselves?

But are we better off than our forefathers? Are we any happier? Have two world wars and the many other conflicts which have taken place, and indeed continue to take place, brought us to our senses? Before reading further, please pause for a long period and think on these things.

You will probably have noticed that *Being in the Way*, the title of this book, is a theme that occurs regularly in many different forms -

helping the young girl on the hospital ship whose mother had died whilst they were in a Japanese prisoner-of-war camp, conducting the evening services during the interregnum at Witley Parish Church and many other instances that form part of my story. 'Being in the way' leads to being in the right place at the right time. I draw your attention again to the biblical narrative in Genesis, chapter 24v27, when Abraham's servant, whilst seeking a wife for his master's son Isaac, meets Rebecca beside the well at Nahor. When the servant realises that God had shown him the woman who is to become Isaac's wife, his words to her are simple, "I, being in the way, the Lord led me".

Lord, for the years

Lord, for the years your love has kept and guided,
Urged and inspired us, cheered us on our way,
Sought us and saved us, pardoned and provided:
Lord of the years, we bring our thanks today.

Lord, for that word, the word of life which fires us,
Speaks to our hearts and sets our souls ablaze,
Teaches and trains, rebukes us and inspires us:
Lord of the word, receive your people's praise.

Lord, for our land, in this our generation,
Spirits oppressed by pleasure, wealth and care:
For young and old, for commonwealth and nation,
Lord of our land, be pleased to hear our prayer.

Lord, for our world, when we disown and doubt him,
Loveless in strength, and comfortless in pain,
Hungry and helpless, lost indeed without him:
Lord of the world, we pray that Christ may reign.

Lord, for ourselves; in living power remake us,
Self on the cross and Christ upon the throne,
Past put behind us, for the future take us:
Lord of our lives, to live for Christ alone.

Timothy Dudley-Smith (b.1926)

Appendices

Appendix 1

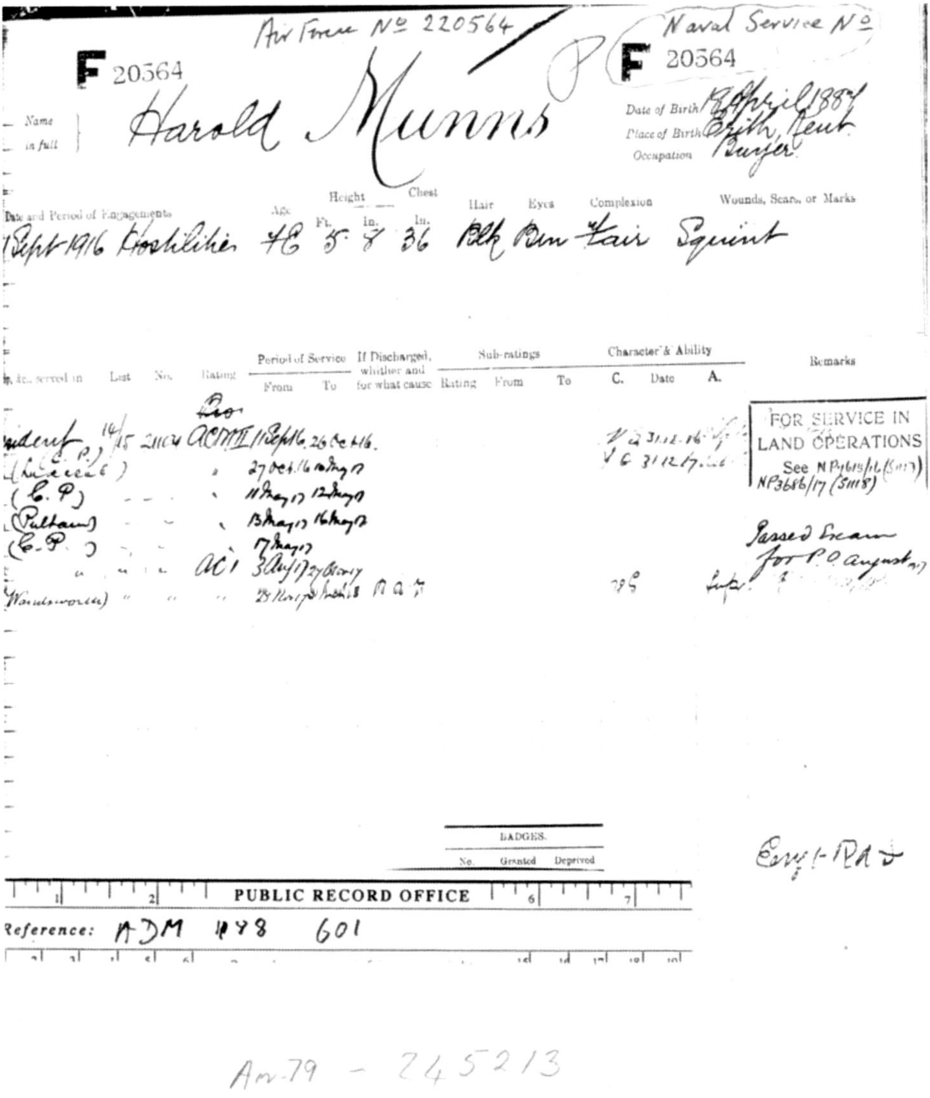
Air Force No 220564

Naval Service No

F 20564

F 20564

Name in full: Harold Munns

Date of Birth: 18 April 1887

Place of Birth: Erith, Kent

Occupation: Buyer

Date and Period of Engagements	Age	Height Ft.	Height In.	Chest In.	Hair	Eyes	Complexion	Wounds, Scars, or Marks
1 Sept 1916 Hostilities	28	5	8	36	Blk	Brn	Fair	Squint

FOR SERVICE IN LAND OPERATIONS See NP1615/16 (5117) NP3686/17 (5118)

Passed Exam for P.O. August 17

BADGES.

PUBLIC RECORD OFFICE

Reference: ADM 188 601

Am-79 – 245213

My Father's Naval Record

Craft No. 6148

When Registered *until 31st March 1911*.
Fee paid £ — : 19 : 11.

Craft Name *Nina*.

Owner's Name *Luke Edward William Munns*.

Owner's Trading Name

Owner's Address *44, Bexley Road, Belvedere, Kent.*
9443.

Description of Craft *Sailing Barge*

Length over all *75 feet* — inches

Width over all amidships after deducting
4 inches for outwales or rubbing pieces *14 ¼ feet* — inches

Depth amidships from under side of deck
or gunwale plank to upper side of ceiling *14 ¼ feet* — inches

Measurement or Registered Tonnage *BY* *38 Tons 14 cwt.*

Weight carrying capacity or Burden Tonnage *64 Tons 18 cwt.*

Permanent Hirer's Name and Address

Other information
February 1924 Registration cancelled — barge not in use since 31 March 1923

Renewed until	Fee paid
31th March 1912	£ — 19 11
31st March 1913	£ — 19 11
31st March 1914	£ — 19 11
31st March 1915	£ — 19 11
31 March 1916	£ — 19 11
31 March 1917	£ — 19 11
31 March 1918	£ — 19 11
31 March 1919	£ — 19 11
31 March 1920	£ — 19 4
31 March 1921	£ — 19 4
31 March 1922	£ — 19 11
31 Mar 1923	£ — 19 4
	£ : :
	£ : :
	£ : :
	£ : :
	£ : :
	£ : :
	£ : :
	£ : :

Registration Certificate - Grandpa's sailing barge *Nina*

Appendix 3

Patent Office Records

Gustave Charles Mohr (Carl Gustav Mohr) - Birmingham, Warwickshire

1864   Patent 2812 - Improvement in cages for birds, squirrels, and other animals.

1868   Patent 2555 - Improvement in the manufacture of cages, baskets, guards, and other articles of wire work.

1869   Patent 2699 - Improvements in the manufacture of cages for birds, squirrels, and other animals.

1873   Patent 2968 - Improvements in the manufacture of metal deed and other boxes, travelling trunks, port manteaus, and similar articles.

1874   Patent 152 - A new or improved method of riveting the joints and seams of deed and other boxes, coal vases, and similar articles.

-?-   Patent 2218 - Improvements in the construction of wire muzzles for dogs and other animals.

1883   Patent 550 - A new and improved spring hasp or clip for securing the lids of trunks, boxes, and the like.

1885   Patent 10,746 - Improvements in the construction & ornamental appearance of bird cages.

1891   Patent 12,062 - Improvements in the construction of muzzles for dogs and other animals (nb. more comfortable for the wearer than 1874 Patent 2218 above).

1897   Patent 5178 - Improvements in the construction of metallic bird cages and other wirework and the piercing tools uses in the manufacture of the same.
Patent 19,339 - Improvement in the construction of gear cases for bicycles, tricycles, and velocipedes. (Registered under the name of Louis Edward Mohr - see patent details in Appendix 4.)

Frederick Edward Mohr – London

1886 Patent 7808 - Combined invalid bed lift, couch, and chair.

1887 Patent 6220 - Improvements in urinals or bed and travelling conveniences for males and females respectively.

Josef Mohr - Vienna, Austria

1857 Patent 2013 - Machinery for propelling vessels.

1896 Patent 21,960 - Improvements in electric bells.

Friedrich Wilhelm Bernhard Mohr – London

1876 Patent 2147 - Improvements in treating spent oxide of iron obtained in the preparation of gas to produce colouring matters and other products.

Carl Mohr, Berlin, Prussia

1877 Patent 398 - Improvements in bottles, jars, and other hollow vessels, and in stoppers for the same, and in machinery for the manufacture of such stoppers.

Hermann Mohr - Mannheim, Germany

1893 Patent 19,926 - Improved suspended weighing machine with steelyard and closed wrought - iron shell.

Theodor Mohr - Cologne, German Empire

1897 Patent 9186 - Improved ventilating boot or shoe.

Max Mohr, Konigsee, Thuringia, Germany

1901 Patent 8279 - Improvements in or relating to newspaper holders and the like.

Appendix 4

19,339 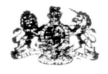 A.D. 1897

Date of Application, 21st Aug., 1897 Complete
Specification Left, 23rd May, 1898—Accepted, 13th Aug., 1898

PROVISIONAL SPECIFICATION,

Improvement in the Construction of Gear Cases for Bicycles, Tricycles, and Velocipedes,

LOUIS ERNEST MOHR, 315, Bolton Road, Small Heath, Birmingham, Metal Worker, do hereby declare the nature of this invention to be as follows: —

The object of this invention is to make a case which only covers the two gear wheels and chain and in no way covers any part of the frame of the bicycle or tricycle.

In order to do this I construct two round boxes with flat sides, each box being in two halves, each half forming a semi-circle, the said halves being connected by means of a hinge.

These round boxes fit over the gear wheels. I connect these two boxes by means of two tubes which completely cover the chain between the gear wheels.

These tubes are soldered on to holes cut in the rim of one of the boxes (the box covering the large gear wheel by preference) where the chain leaves the gear wheel.

Holes are cut in the rim of the small box where the chain leaves the gear wheel and on these I solder short tubes.

So that the small box may pass the chain I cut a slot through the rim and through the short tubes, the slot being afterwards closed with a slide fitting in grooves in the sides of the box.

As an outlet for any waste lubricating matter I cut a hole in the bottom of the case, the said hole being covered by a slide.

To adjust the case I detach the chain, thread it through the tubes on the large box, place it in position over the gear wheels and fasten the connecting link of the chain.

I then take the small box, close it over the small gear wheel and fix the slide in the slot.

Dated this 20th day of August 1897.

LOUIS ERNEST MOHR

Impt. in the Construction of Gear Cases for Bicycles, Tricycles, and Velocipedes.

same is to be performed, to be particularly described and ascertained in and by the following statement:—

The object of this invention is to make a case which only covers the two gear wheels and chain, and in no way covers any part of the frame of the bicycle or tricycle, and also to make a case which is practically dust-proof.

In order to do this I construct two round boxes with flat sides, each box being in two halves, each half forming a semi-circle, said halves being connected by means of a hinge. These round boxes fit over the gear wheels.

I connect these two boxes by means of two tubes which completely cover the chain between the gear wheels. These tubes are permanently fixed on to holes cut in the rim of one of the boxes (the box covering the large gear wheel by preference) where the chain leaves the gear wheel.

Holes are cut in the rim of the small box where the chain leaves the gear wheel, and on these I fix short tubes.

So that the small box may pass the chain I cut a slot through the rim and through the short tubes, the slot being afterwards closed with a slide fitting in grooves in the sides of the box.

As an outlet for any excess of lubricating matter I cut a hole in the bottom of the case, said hole being covered by a slide. To adjust the case I detach the chain, thread it through the tubes (Fig. A 1 and A 2) on the large box (Fig. B 1 and B 2), place it in position over the gear wheels (Fig. 1 drawing left with the Provisional Specification) and fasten the connecting link of the chain.

I then take the small box (Letter C), close it over the small gear wheel (Fig. 2 drawing left with the Provisional Specification) and fix the slide (letter D drawing left with the Provisional Specification) in the slot (letter G drawing left with the Provisional Specification).

It has been found more convenient to hinge the small box (letter C) at such an angle as to allow the top tube on the large box (Fig. A 1) to rest on the bottom half of the small box (letter C) when the case is closed (at the points marked letter E, drawing left with the Complete Specification) and sliding the bottom tube on the small box (letter F) over the bottom tube on the large box (Fig. A 2), thus allowing the chain to be threaded through the tubes on the large box and through the bottom half of the small box (drawing left with the Complete Specification).

Having now particularly described and ascertained the nature of my said invention, and in what manner the same is to be performed, I declare that what I claim is:—

Constructing a gear case for bicycles, tricycles, and velocipedes of two round boxes with flat sides, each box being halved and connected by means of a hinge, and two tubes completely covering the chain, between the gear wheels, the tubes being permanently fixed on to one of the boxes (the box covering the large gear wheel by preference), the said box being hinged in such a manner as to allow the chain being slid through both tubes and box when the case is open.

Dated this 19th day of May 1898.

L. E. MOHR.

Redhill : Printed for Her Majesty's Stationery Office, by Malcomson & Co., Ltd.—1898

A.D. 1897. Aug. 21. N°. 19,339.
MOHR'S Provisional Specification.

(1 SHEET)

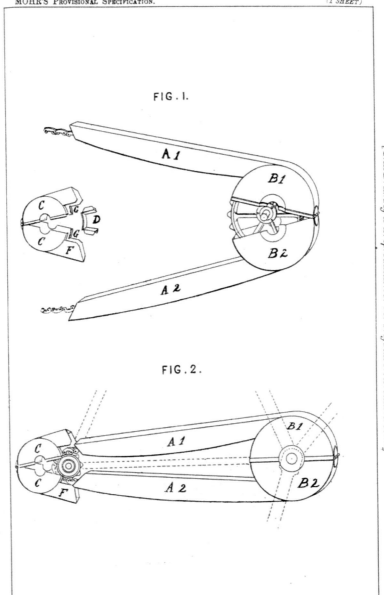

FIG.1.

FIG.2.

[This Drawing is a reproduction of the Original on a reduced scale.]

A.D. 1897. Aug. 21. Nº 19,339.
MOHR'S Complete Specification.

(1 SHEET)

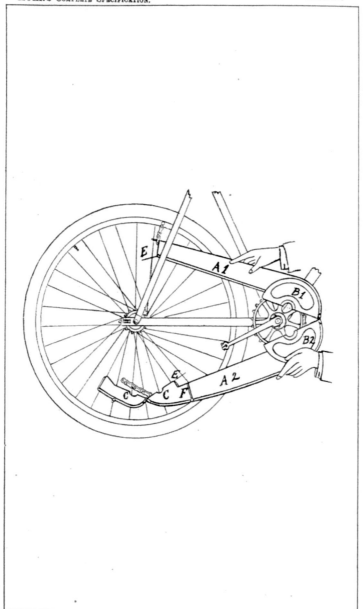

Malby &Sons. Photo-Litho.

Appendix 5

The Prussian *Kriegsdenkmunze* (war memorial medal), which was made in various forms with different dates on it (see the two photos attached). The medal was made from the bronze of captured guns, and that is what the lettering around the edge of it says: "aus erobertem Geschiitz". The words on the back (!) under the crown and cypher are "PreuBens tapfern Kriegern" (to Prussia's brave warriors), the inscription around the medal is "Gott war mit uns, Ihm sey die Ehre!" (God was with us, give him the honour). The wreath and dates on the front (!) are within the Prussian iron cross, which is well known.

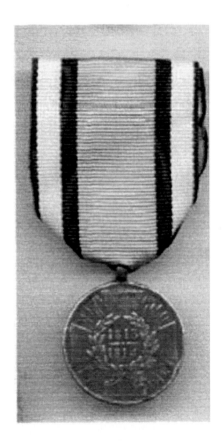

Prussian War Memorial Medal

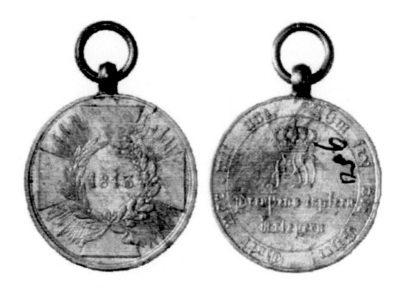

Prussian Army Medal

Appendix 6

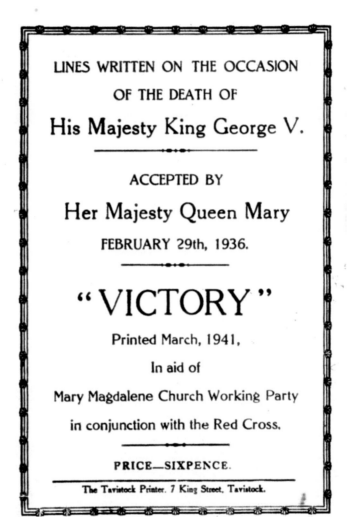

LINES WRITTEN ON THE OCCASION
OF THE DEATH OF

His Majesty King George V.

ACCEPTED BY

Her Majesty Queen Mary

FEBRUARY 29th, 1936.

" VICTORY "

Printed March, 1941,

In aid of

Mary Magdalene Church Working Party

in conjunction with the Red Cross.

PRICE—SIXPENCE.

The Tavistock Printer. 7 King Street, Tavistock.

Auntie Ethel's poem

VICTORY

The fight is o'er, the battle won
King George has laid his weapons down;
And God has called to him - Well done;
Come and wear a Holy Crown.

All nations mourn, his Empire weep,
Their King has gone to rest.
For God has given eternal sleep
To him whom He hath blest.

His noble life, through years of strife
Has won a nations heart.
Supported by his faithful wife,
He manfully took his part.

An Empire free from sin and woe
Was his great hope in life.
So may his people onward go
And cease this endless strife.

If King George could only speak.
This is what he would say:
Bid my Empire not to weep
But work for the crowning day.

When wars shall cease and God shall claim
His Kingship of the World,
And He shall loose the captives' chains
And Satans' host be furled.

When the King of Kings is crowned.
And claims His long lost sheep.
King George may see his Empire found
Ready their King to meet.

Composed by:-
Ethel M. Mohr,
Jan. 28th, 1936

Appendix 7

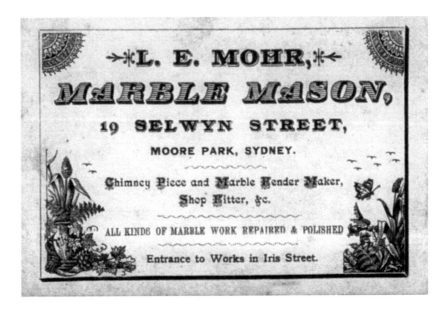

Grandfather's business card c.1883

Appendix 8

Bibliography

An Investigation and Recommendations concerning the Future of Dentistry
Joint Planning Committee of Dental Students
October 1942

****

Large Dental Cyst of Right Maxilla
Douglas Munns Surg/Lt. (D), RNVR
D. Gaz. 11.26 Sept. 1944.

****

Presentation for Teaching of the Operation of Gingivectomy
Douglas Munns
Brit. D. J. 87:295-297. Dec. 2, 1949.

****

Malocclusion: its aetiology and principles of treatment
Douglas Munns
Brit. D. J. 89:209-211. Nov. 7, 1950.

****

Gingivectomy Splint
Douglas Munns
Brit. D. J. 92:184-185. April 1, 1952.

****

Development of the Dental Department in a General Hospital since the Introduction of the NHS
Douglas Munns, VRD
Brit. D. J. 107323. Dec. 1, 1959.

****

Impacted Second Mandibular Molars
Douglas Munns
Dental Practitioner. 1959 Vol. X, No. 2

****

A Case of Partial Anodontia and Supernumerary Tooth Present in the Same Jaw
Dental Practitioner & Dental Record. 18(1):34-7,
Sept 1967

****

A Metallurgical Examination of Fractured Stainless-Steel Wire in Orthodontic Appliances.
Harcourt, H. J., Munns, D.
Dental Practitioner and Dental Record. 17(9):307-12.
May 1967

****

An Analysis of Broken Removable Appliances
Munns, D.
Transactions of the British Society for the Study of Orthodontics.
57:45-8, 1970-71

****

Administration of the Dental Health Services of England 1907-1978.

Dental Practice (Epsom)
July to October 1979

****

Unerupted Incisors
Munns, D.
British Journal of Orthodontics
8(1):39-42, Jan 1981

****

The First Twenty-five Years
Christian Dental Fellowship

****

The British Society of Peridontology – the First Fifty Years
Letter from Douglas Munns – page 45.
Published 1999

****

Appendix 9

Acknowledgements

A History of the Royal Dental Hospital of London and School of Dental Surgery 1885 -1985

Ernest Smith & Beryl Cottell
The Athlone Press. ISBN 0-485-11517-4

****

A Short History of St. George's Hospital and Origins of its Ward Names

Terry Gould & David Uttley
ISBN 0-485-11504-2 and 0-485-12126-3

****

A History of Atkinson Morley's Hospital 1869-1995

Terry Gould & David Uttley
0-485-11515-0 and 0-485-12126-5

****

Deep Sea Diving and Submarine Operation – 6th Edition

Sir Robert Davis
Siebe, Gorman & Co. Ltd., Cwmbran, Gwent.

****

History of London Underground – Hammersmith to Finsbury Park

****

Underwater Medicine

Stanley Miles & D.E. Mackay

****

The War of Invention- Scientific Developments 1914 – 1918

Guy Hartcup
Brassey's Defence Publishers

****

The First Air War

T.C. Treadwell & Alan C. Wood
Brassey – 1996

****

Barnes & Mortlake Past with East Sheen

Massie Brown
Historical Publications Ltd. (1997)

****

A History of Mortlake

The Anderson Series
E & E Plumridge Ltd. (1983)

****

Spritsail Barges of the Thames and Medway

Edward J. Marsh
Percival Marshall (1948)

****

Men of the Tideway

Dick Fagan & Eric Burgess
Robert Hale – London – 1966.

****

The Journal of the Rev John Wesley, AM
Vols. I-IV

Vol. I 1730 – 1743
Vol. II 1746 – 1760
J.M. Dent & Sons Ltd., 1906

****

The Night Blitz 1940 – 1941

John Ray
Arms and Armour Press, 1996

****

Witness to the Word
(A History of Oak Hill College, 1932 – 2000)

Rudolph Heinze & David Wheaton
Paternoster Press 2002

****

The City of London School

A.E. Douglas-Smith
Basil Blackwell, 1937. Oxford

****

Harringay Story
The official record of the Billy Graham Greater London Crusade 1954

Frank Colquhoun
Hodder & Stoughton, London

****

Sermons by the Rev William Braden
(Late minister of Kings's Weigh House Chapel, City of London)

Edited by Agnes Braden
James Clarke & Co. 1880, London

****

Guide to Tracing Your Ancestors (Debrett's Guide)

Noel Carrer-Briggs & Royston Gantier
Webb & Dower, 1981

****

County librarians, archivists, and other staff in Birmingham, Buckinghamshire, City of London, City of Westminster, Devon, Kent and Surrey.

Family Records Offices, National Archives and numerous national libraries throughout the United Kingdom, Australia and Austria.

Various Family History Societies (FHS), particularly Anglo-German FHS and North Kent FHS.

Eastbourne Tourism.

Appendix 10

Clergy of the Church of England, now deceased or retired, who have influenced my life over the years

(From information given in: *Crockford's Clerical Directory*, The Church Commissioner's of England and The Central Board of Finance of the Church of England)

Canon Richard William Frederick WOOTTON - 'Dick'

Corpus Christie College, Oxford
      1st Class Cl. Mods. 1934
      1st Class Lit. Hum. 1936
      BA 1939
      MA 1939
Missionary with CMS India 1937 onwards
Red Cross Commissioner, India and Far East 1941-46
MBE 1946
Wycliffe Hall, Oxford - 1946
Dip. Th. 1947
      Deacon - 1947 Diocese of London
      Priested- 1948 Diocese of Lahore
Priest-in-charge, Gojra Mission 1948-57
Principal, St. John's Divinity School, Narowal 1952-53
Tutor Gujrambzala Theological Seminary 1953-6
Hon.Canon, Lahore from 1958
Principal, Church Army Training College 1961-66
Assistant Translations Secretary, British & Foreign Bible Society.
                                    1966-69

Deputy Translations Secretary, BFBS 1969-70
Secretary, BFBS 1970-73
Lecturer of St. John Baptist, Knighton 1973-80
Chaplain for Community Relations, Diocese of Leicester 1974 – 80
Licensed to officiate, Diocese of Sarum, from 1981

Rev. George Adolphous Samuel ADAMS

Rustat Scholar - Jesus College, Cambridge - BA (Aegrot
Maths. Tripos) - 1881
MA - 1889

Wells College - 1881
Curate, Weston-super Mare, 1881-18 84.
Chaplain,. Rosanio de Santa Fe, 1884-1893
Vicar, Erith, Kent, 1894-1917
Rector, Nettlestead (Rochester), 1917- ?

Rev. Jack Arthur Gibson AINLEY

Jesus College, Cambridge -   BA 1914
MA 1919

Ridley Hall, Cambridge
Deacon 1919
Priested 1920
Curate, New Sheldon, 1919-1922
Melcombe Regis - 1922-24
Vicar, Christ Church, Lowestoft, 1924-28
St. Paul's, Cambridge, 1928-1937
Rector, Morden, 1937- ?
Patron, Camford School Ltd

Rev. Herbert Walter BENSON.

(Mortlake Parish Church - Baptism)
Emmanuel Collage, Cambrdge - MA
Curate, St. Mary's, Paddington, 1914-1916
Curate, St. Mary's, Mortlake, 1916-

Rev. Philip Thomas Charles CASE (Witley Parish Church)

B.Sc Economics (London) 1951
Sarum Theological College - 1951
Deacon - 1953
Priested - 1954
Curate, Westminster St. Stephens & St. John's London, 1953-56

Curate, St. Mathews, Ashford (Middx), 1956-58
Curate-in-Charge, Ashford (Middx) St. Hilda, 1958-61
Vicar, St. Hillier (Southwark), 1961-66
Vicar, Witley (Guildford), 1966-84
Rural Dean, Godalming, 1979-84
Retired 1984

Canon Jack Joseph CRESSWELL (Busbridge Church)
Queens College, Cambridge,   BA 1939
                                                    MA 1943
Wycliffe Hall, Oxford, 1939
            Deacon - 1940
            Priested - 1941
Curate, St. Helens, St. Helens (Liverpool) 1940-46
Vicar, Iver (Oxford), 1946-56
Rector, Windlesham (Guildford), 1956-62
Vicar, Horsell (Guildford), 1962-70
Hon. Canon, Guildford Cathedral, 1969-78
Rector, Busbridge (Guildford), 1970-78
Retired 1978

Rev. Cecil Howard Dunsten CULLINGFORD
(Commandant Varsity & Public School. North Wales VP.S Camp -
1933-35)
Late scholar - Christ Church College, Cambridge
            1st Class Classical Tripos - Pt.i.   1925 BA, Pt. ii. 1926
            1st Class History Tripos - Pt. ii. 1927
                                                    MA 1930
Clifton Theological College - 1932-1934
            Deacon – 1933
            Priested - 1934
            Vice-Principal 1932-193
Assistant Chaplain, Oundle School, 1933-1934
Chaplain, Oundle School, 1935
Chaplain to the Forces, 1939-45.
Headmaster, Monmouth School, 1946-

Rev. George Bailie DUNCAN

Dob. 1912

Travelling secretary, Scripture Union, 1934 - 1937

Deacon - 1937

Priested - 1938

Curate – St. James', Carlisle, 1937 - 1938

Minister, a church in Edinburgh - 1938-51

Incumbant, Christ Church, Cockfosters (Ecclesiastical
                              Conventional District), 1951-58

Minister in Church of Scotland, 1958 onwards

Canon Bertram Cecil HOPSON

Calcutta University - BA 1904

Ridley Hall, Cambridge 1905

        Deacon – 1906

        Priested - 1907

Curate, St. Andrews-the-less, Cambridge, 1906-1908

        All Saints, Eastbourne, 1909-1912

Vicar, Christ Church, Trent Park, Cockfosters, 1912-1949

Temp. Chaplain to the forces, 1917-1920

Hon. Chaplain to the forces from 1920

Died December 1949

Rev. Leonard George JANES

Keeble College, Oxford -   BA 1939

                              MA - 1943

Ely Theological College – 1939

        Deacon 1941

        Priested 1942

Curate, Withycombe Raleigh, 1941 -43

Chaplain RNVR, 1943

        HMHS Gerusalemme, 1945-1947

Curate, Cowley, Oxford, 1947-1950

Priest-in-charge, Abingdon, 1950-1956

Vicar, St. Barnabas, Oxford, 1956-1960

Chaplain, HM Prison, Exeter, 1960-67.
Permission to officiate, Diocese of Brisbane, 1967-1968
Permission to officiate, Diocese of Oxford, 1968-

Rt. Rev. Leslie Albert KNIGHT - Bishop of Bunbury, Western Australia

University of New Zealand,   BA 1913
                             MA 1914
University of London,Board of Theological Studies iv parti.
                             Th.L. 1915
        Deacon 1914
        Preisted 1915
Curate, Fendalton,1914-1916
Priest-in-charge, Malvern with Honorata, 1916-1917
Chaplain to New Zealand Expeditionary Force, 1919-1921
Warden of St. Barnabas Theological Coll. (with Cathedral appointments at Adelaide), 1928-1938
Inducted as Bishop of Bunbury in St. George's Cathedral, Perth, 25th January 1938

Preb. Donald Macleod LYNCH

Late Scholar of Pembroke College, Cambs.
        1st class Tripos, pt.i. 1932
                    pt. li 1934
                    BA 1934
                    MA 1937
Wycliffe Hall. Oxford, 1934
        Deacon 1935
        Priested 1936
Curate, Christ Church, Chelsea, 1935-38
Tutor, Oakhill Theological Coll. 1938-40
Curate, St. Michael & All Angels, Stonebridge Park, 1940-42
Minister of All Souls, Queensbury, London, 1942-50
Vicar, St. Luke's Tunbridge Wells, 1950-53
Principal of Church Army Training College, 1953-61
Chief Secretary, Church Army, 1960-76

Preb. of Twyford in St. Paul's Cathedral from 1964
Chaplain to HM The Queen from 1969
OBE 1972
Curate-in-charge, St. Lawrence, Send, 1976

Rev. Herbert A. MAIS
G & C College, Cambridge, BA 1884

MA 1890

Curate, Branksome, Dorset, 1885-1887
        Stoke Bridge, Glos., 1887-1890
        Ifield, Sussex, 1890-1897
Vicar, Stanley with Horton, 1897-1901
Rector, Egdean, 1901-1903
Vicar, Burpham, Surrey, 1903-1913
        Cold, Waltham, 1913-1917
Assistant Clergy, Mortlake with East Sheen, 1917-

Rev. John Esward MATTHEWS
University College, North Wales, BA 1910
Curate, St. Mary the Virgin, Cardiff, 1911-1913
        Howarden, 1913-1921
        Christ Church, Chester, 1921-22
        St. John, Bebbington, 1922-1924
Priest-in-charge, Gretna with Eastriggs, 1924-1926
Curate, Ramsey, 1926-1929
        Thames Ditton, 1929-1934
Vicar, All Saints, Weston, Thames Ditton, 1934-1937
Vicar, Christ Church, Epsom Common, 1937-

Rev. Albert Edward ROBINS
University of London - BA 1924
Bishops College, Cheshunt, 1929
Curate, St. Martin's, Dorking, 1930-1935
        All Saints, Weston (in charge of Hinchley Wood), 1935-
                                                           1939
Curate-in-charge, Hinchley Wood conventional district, 1939-

Rev. Edward Heathfield TUPPER

St. Edmund's Hall, Oxford -   BA 1899
                              MA 1903

Ely College - 1901
Curate, Wantage, 1902-1906
Worcester Cathedral - Minor Canon, 1906-1908
                       Sacrist,1908-1918
                       Precentor, 1909-1918
Vicar, Mortlake with East Sheen, 1918

Preb. Stephen Mortimer WARNER

University College, Durham - BA 1894
                              M.A. 1899
London College of Divinity- 1894
        Deacon 1896
        Priested 1897
Curate, St. Simon's, Southsea, 1896-1898
Vicar, Severnake, 1898-1900
        St. Paul, Poole, 1900-1901
        All Saints, Plumstead, 1901-1910
        Sandown, I.O.W., 1910-1914
        St. Paul, Peng, 1914-1919
Temporary RN Chaplain, 1917-1919
Vicar, Holy Trinity, Eastbourne, 1919-1947
Preb. Chichester (Ipthorne), 1930
Proc. Conv. from 1931

Walter Harold YEANDLE

New College, Oxford -   BA 1922
                              MA 1924
Wells Theological College – 1924
        Deacon,1924
        Priested 1925

Curate Mortlake with East Sheen, 1924-1931
        Thornbury-on-Tees, 1936-37
Curate in charge, St. Chads Conventional District, Middlesburgh, 1937-44
Vicar, Bearsted, Dioc. of Canterbury, 1944 to 19__ (no entry
                                                    after 1952)

Also to note:
Rev. John MUNNS, Raddenhall, Norfolk - 1703
Rev. C. Oliver MUNNS, Bath - 1876
Rev. Peter Thomas MUNNS - 1952/53
Rev. Stuart MUNNS - 1960/61

Appendix 11

Development of the Dental Department in a General Hospital since the Introduction of the National Health Service

Douglas Munns L.D.S.
Highlands General Hospital

As the completion of the first decade of the National Health Service coincided with the annual conference of the Association in Dundee, it was thought that a review of the organisation of a dental department of a hospital within the service would be of interest to members. Consequently, some research into the matter was undertaken and the result presented in the form of a demonstration, and it is this that forms the basis of this paper. (Owing to delay in printing this paper, graphs and tables have been modified to include 1958 records.)

This hospital was built at the close of the last century as a fever hospital and remained as such under London County Council authority until the beginning of the last war; dental treatment was therefore provided by the council's dental staff. During the 1939-1945 war, it became a sector hospital under the Emergency Medical Service and a visiting dental surgeon was appointed to the staff. At the close of the war, it gradually changed its nature and at the commencement of the National Health Service in July 1948, it consisted mainly of chronic sick, there being some 250 post-encephalitis lethargic (PEL) patients and 100 tuberculosis patients, and a dental surgeon attended twice weekly; there was a small dental room with adequate equipment for routine dental treatment, although exodontias and prosthetics constituted much of the work.

From 1948 onwards, the nature of the hospital has changed considerably. Today we have some 230 acute beds with consultants in most specialities holding regular sessions at the hospital, and there are modern twin operating theatres, pathology laboratory, etc.; owing to the decline in tuberculosis there are now only ten beds for chest cases, and, through natural courses, the number of PEL patients is on the decline; graph (fig. 1) illustrates this. The dental surgeon is also responsible for patients at a small practitioner hospital of 52 acute beds, a geriatric hospital of 88 beds, and a small recovery hospital.

233

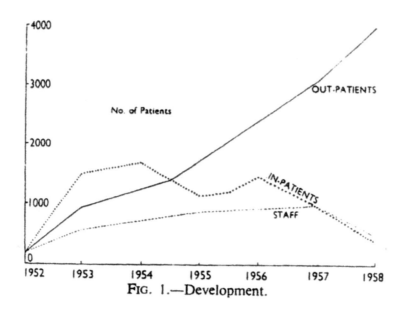

FIG. 1.—Development.

Through the foresight of the regional board's Dental Advisory Committee and the co-operation of the management committee and medical superintendent, plans were made soon after the introduction of the National Health Service for a small bungalow-type building to be allocated as a dental department, and for a full-time senior hospital dental officer, dental technicians and other ancillary staff to be appointed. It was not until September 1951 that the full-time SHDO was appointed and the new dental department was opened in April 1952 and, with the alterations and modifications that have been made since then, fig. 2 shows a plan of the present department. The two dental surgeries are each of 130 sq. ft. in area and equipped with Sterling Junior units to enable special conservative, exodontias, and other operative procedures to be undertaken under local anaesthetic. The fact that there are two surgeries facilitates a greater turnover of patients and also enables a hygienist to be employed. At the moment, there is one dental surgery assistant and one state-enrolled nurse, both part-time to the department; unfortunately, this hospital, like so many others, is so short of nursing staff that it is not possible to make a fully trained nurse available to the department. The dental laboratory is 200 sq. ft. in area and the equipment, over and above the usual laboratory equipment, includes an electric oven, centrifugal casting machine,

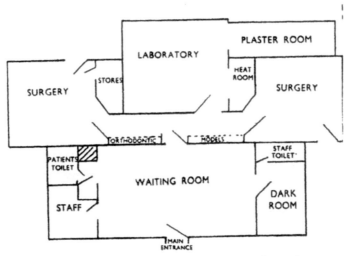

FIG. 2.—Plan of Department. Scale ⅓" = 5'.

and electronic welder. As well as routine prostheses, chrome-cobalt and nylon dentures, surgical prostheses and many orthodontic appliances are constructed both for this hospital and the Royal Northern Hospital. There are now two dental technicians employed, a senior surgical technician and a senior technician, the latter almost entirely engaged in the construction of orthodontic appliances. It will thus be seen that this department conforms very closely to the recommendations of the BDA in their recent report (1957) with the exception that no X-ray apparatus is installed in the department. Whilst agreeing that such apparatus would have many advantages I am afraid that if it were installed, the hospital radiologist would expect us to take all the dental radiographs. The time involved would considerably reduce the number of patients that could be seen by the dental surgeon.

The Ministry of Health, in their booklet "Hospital Dental Service" (1954) state:

"(1) *General.* Persons requiring dental treatment and appliances under the National Health Service will normally avail themselves of the arrangements made with dental practitioners by the executive councils, i.e. the general dental services provided under Part IV of the Act, or if they are in the 'priority' classes (expectant and nursing mothers and children,) of the service organised by local health and educational authorities. It is not, therefore, a function of the hospital service, apart from the special case of dental hospitals, to provide a dental service for the general public; but it is an essential part of the service to make the necessary arrangement for:

    i. the dental care of long-stay hospital in-patients;

    ii the dental care of out-patients and short-stay in-patients for whom such care is a necessary part of their hospital treatment;

    iii The provision of consultant advice and treatment for cases of special difficulty referred to hospitals by general dental practitioners.

(2) For long-stay hospital in-patients, the aim should be to provide facilities for full conservative dental treatment and not merely for extractions.

(3) In addition for provision for routine dental care, a suitable number of hospital beds should be provided for patients needing major dental operative treatment.

The following table shows the percentages of patients treated during 1957:

	Per cent
Long-stay in-patients	21
Out-patients and short-stay in-patients requiring treatment as a necessary part of their hospital treatment	. 11
Patients referred by general dental practitioners as requiring consultant advice or as cases of special difficulty 52	

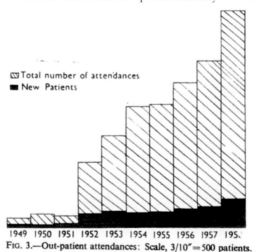

Fig. 3.—Out-patient attendances: Scale, 3/10″=500 patients.

A glance at the graph (fig. 1) and also the out-patients table (fig. 3) will show how more and more local dental practitioners are making use of the consultants hospital service. Two other categories of patients also receive treatment:

(1) Those referred from the Casualty Department of the hospital, but here it has to be remembered that these must not be 'toothache' cases, which are the responsibility of the general dental practitioner and not of the hospital service.

(2) Members of the medical, nursing, and lay staff of the hospital, but there again, such treatment is to be regarded as a 'privilege' rather than a 'right', and as other patients increase, there will be less time available to treat staff.

During the year 1957, 3 per cent of total patient treatments were referred from Casualty Department and 13 per cent were staff.

There are two main divisions of work of any hospital dental officer; time spent in the operating theatre and time spent in the dental surgery or on ward rounds, although one must never lose sight of the importance of research which should always be in the forefront of his duties. There are now three beds provided for patients needing dental operative treatment and one session per week (other than emergencies) is spent in the operating theatre and a glance at fig.4 will show how the demand has gradually increased over the past few years. The following is an analysis of operations performed during 1957:

				Per cent
Abnormalities of dentition	..			9
Apicectomies	..	..	..	4
Impacted teeth	..	..	..	48
Neoplasms ..	..	..	..	7
Retained roots	..	..	..	12
Routine extractions		..	..	20

A comparison of the 1957 and 1958 records is of interest, and, taking into account all categories of patients who received treatment in the dental surgery (i.e. excluding those referred to in the previous paragraph), our records show that out of the total number of patents seen, treatments were given as follows:

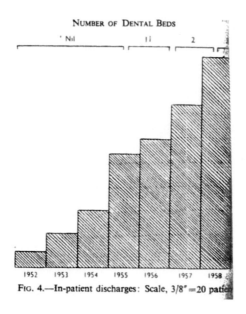

NUMBER OF DENTAL BEDS

Nil · · · 1½ · · · 2

1952 1953 1954 1955 1956 1957 1958

FIG. 4.—In-patient discharges: Scale, 3/8″ =20 patients

		1957	1958
		Per cent	Per cent
Conservative	..	11	5
Orthodontic	..	26	52
Peridontal	..	22	9
Prosthetic	..	6	2
Surgical	..	16	18
Radiographs	..	55	60

The decline in conservative and prosthetic treatments provided is only a reflection of the fact that, owing to the increase in the number of out-patients referred to the department, it has been possible to treat only a few staff during the year.

Experience has shown that there is a great need for a hospital orthodontic service as many general dental practitioners are not prepared to accept cases under the National Health Service, and, in this area at any rate, there is a very long waiting list in the School Dental Service; it is therefore not surprising that many such cases are referred to this hospital and receive treatment. The above figures show the value of this speciality within the hospital service.

No paper of this nature would be complete without reference to two important aspects of the work of a hospital dental officer. Whereas the general dental practitioner only sees perhaps one interesting case in the course of a year, the hospital dental officer has many such cases coming to his clinics. It is therefore his duty to see that those members of the profession who are in a less fortunate position than he is, have an opportunity to advance their knowledge by learning about some of these cases, and it is therefore imperative that such facilities should be given. In this area it has now become the custom to arrange a clinical meeting as one of the regular meetings of the local branch of the association and this is held in this hospital, when such cases are presented. Secondly, every member of the profession should be interested instructing the public in oral hygiene and such centres as hospitals and schools are ideal places where visual aids can be used. For several years, therefore, we have at least once a year and sometimes more often, invited all our dental out-patients to view one or more of the oral hygiene films that are available, and we have found that these have always been much appreciated and evoked many questions.

Since this survey was written in 1958, a report on the consultant dental service in the Birmingham area has been presented by Hales (1959). This approaches the subject from a different angle and gives a picture of the work of a consultant in a fully established department rather than the build-up of a new dental department in a general hospital; further, in Birmingham there is also an orthodontic consultant service.

I must agree with Hales on the question of an appointment system for, whilst no patient in pain must be kept waiting for any long period of time (quite often relief can be easily given by their own general dental practitioner whilst waiting for an appointment at the hospital), it is quite possible and desirable to see all patients by appointment and thus avoid unnecessary time at the hospital waiting to see the consultant. Naturally one has the odd emergency, which can cause chaos to the rest of the session, but difficulties occur very frequently and if one has a spare surgery available it is usually possible to keep the emergency under observation whilst proceeding with the booked patients. Indeed, one is bound to conclude that the expansion of the consultative dental service is urgently necessary.

In conclusion, I must express my thanks to the management committee in placing material at my disposal to enable me to prepare this paper, and also to the staff of this hospital, especially those in the Dental Department, who have spent many hours in tabulating records on my behalf.

REFERENCES

"Hospital Dental Service (1954) Ministry of Health HM (54) 94.
"The Development of the Hospital Dental Service – conditions and minimum requirements required to provide a satisfactory service" (1957) BDA Hospitals Group.
HALES, W.B. (1959) *Dent. Mag. (Lond.)*, 76, 73.

British Dental Journal vol. 107, 1959

Family Trees